Attention Deficit Hyperactivity Disorder Handbook

T0189968

J. Gordon Millichap

Attention Deficit Hyperactivity Disorder Handbook

A Physician's Guide to ADHD

Second Edition

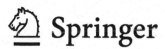

J. Gordon Millichap, MD
Pediatric Neurologist
Children's Memorial Hospital
Northwestern University Medical School
Chicago, Illinois
USA

ISBN 978-1-4419-1396-8 (hardcover)   ISBN 978-1-4419-1397-5 (eBook)
ISBN 978-1-4614-2021-7 (softcover)
DOI 10.1007/978-1-4419-1397-5
Springer New York Heidelberg Dordrecht London

Library of Congress Control Number: 2009938108

Printed on acid-free paper

Springer is part of Springer Science+Business Media (www.springer.com)

In tribute to Nancy, and to Martin, Paul, Gordon, and John

Preface

ADHD, or attention deficit hyperactivity disorder, is a syndrome commonly encountered in children and adolescents, and occasionally in adults. It is often associated with learning disabilities, resulting in failure to achieve the expected level of academic performance. At least one child in every classroom and approximately 3–5% of the school-age population is inattentive, hyperactive, or both. The cause is diverse and often undetermined; genetic and environmental factors are invoked. A family member, either parent or sibling, has a history of ADHD in an estimated 80%, and minor anomalies of brain development, premature birth and anoxic injury, infection, and toxic nicotine and lead exposure are some of the presumed causes. A neurological basis for ADHD is supported by reports of MRI evidence of structural brain abnormalities, electroencephalographic dysrhythmias, and subtle signs of immature brain development on neurological examination.

Parents may recognize hyperactive behavior soon after birth or when the child begins to walk, but the diagnosis is frequently delayed until a teacher observes the inability to focus, distractibility, and restless behavior in the classroom. An initial evaluation by the pediatrician or family physician is usually followed by consultations with the pediatric neurologist or psychiatrist, a psychological evaluation, and laboratory investigations when indicated.

Treatment consists of educational accommodations, medications, behavior modification, and family counseling. Central nervous stimulants have a remarkable beneficial effect in 80% of ADHD children, helping them to focus, reducing distractibility and restless behavior, and facilitating learning and memory. Used in conservative doses, as an aid to education, and monitored closely by a physician, stimulant medications are free from serious side effects. Alternative therapies, including diet, and visual and auditory training, may be supportive but rarely have the immediate and measurable effects of pharmacotherapy.

This book is written for the practicing pediatrician, and residents and fellows in pediatrics, pediatric neurology, neurology, and psychiatry. The psychologist, social worker, therapist, the interested teacher and student, and concerned and informed parents should also find the book of value. This *Attention Deficit Hyperactivity Disorder Handbook* is an expanded professional, updated edition and revision, incorporating advances in the last decade. More than one hundred new references, many related to causes and treatment of ADHD, are included. Questions most frequently asked by parents and teachers who care for the child with attention deficit and related disorders are addressed. The methods of management and selection of medications are supported when possible by published reports of controlled studies. References are listed for all publications.

The reader should be able to evaluate the current extent of our knowledge of diagnosis, treatment methods, and outcome of children with ADHD. It is hoped that the book will lead to a better understanding of the child with ADHD and improvement in the medical, educational, and psychological management.

Chicago, Illinois   J. Gordon Millichap, M.D., F.R.C.P.

Acknowledgments

My patients, many of whom have overcome or compensated for their attention deficits and are leading successful adult lives, and their parents, who nurture and support them through difficult times, are the inspiration for this book. My associate, nurse practitioner Michelle Yee, who shares the challenge and satisfaction in caring for and helping our patients to achieve in school. Colleagues in pediatrics and other medical disciplines, who refer patients for neurological evaluation. The teachers, who facilitate and monitor their students' responses to therapy. The psychologists, who evaluate and provide child and family counseling, without which the medical management of our patients would be incomplete. My friend, Dr. Terry Finn and son, Martin Millichap, who read the manuscript and made helpful suggestions regarding the psychologist's role in the management of ADHD. My sons, Paul, Gordon and Dr. John Millichap, who advised on various aspects of the project, and my late wife, Nancy, teacher and author of a book on dyslexia, who encouraged me to continue an interest in attention deficit and learning disorders.

I am indebted to all.

J. Gordon Millichap

Contents

Chapter 1
Definition and History of ADHD

ADHD, the abbreviation for *Attention-Deficit/Hyperactivity Disorder*, is the name coined to describe children, adolescents, and some adults, who are inattentive, easily distracted, abnormally overactive, and impulsive in their behavior. ADHD is a neurobiological "syndrome," not a "disease," with a specific known cause. Many different factors have been suggested as the cause of ADHD. The treatment requires several different approaches, involving medical, neuropsychological, educational, and parental disciplines. It is a "heterogeneous" disorder.

Under different names, ADHD has been recognized for more than a century. It is not a new diagnosis or a reflection of this twentieth century, competitive and fast-moving society. In the nineteenth century, Heinrich Hoffman (1809–1874), a German physician and poet, wrote about Fidgety, Philip, 1955 who could not sit still. The poem portrays the typical behavior of a child with ADHD, living in times when children were subject to discipline less permissive than at present. A stricter control of behavior did not appear to prevent the occurrence of the hyperkinetic syndrome.

Brain Damage Syndromes

Medical reference to a similar childhood behavioral syndrome dates back to the beginning of the twentieth century, in articles published in the British journal, *Lancet* (1902, 1904) and the *Journal of the American Medical Association* (1921). Behavioral abnormalities were associated with head injury in the earliest reports, and they occurred as a complication of encephalitis following the World War I influenza epidemic of 1918.

The similarities of the hyperkinetic behavior following head trauma and that described in children recovering from encephalitis were described in later articles (Hohman, 1922; Ebaugh, 1923; Strecker and Ebaugh, 1924). These authors found the children distractible as well as overactive. "Organic drivenness" was a term used to describe the behavioral disturbance following epidemic encephalitis, and damage to the brainstem was suggested as the underlying cause (Kahn and Cohen, 1934). This description of behavioral symptoms caused by brain disease or

J.G. Millichap, *Attention Deficit Hyperactivity Disorder Handbook*,
DOI 10.1007/978-1-4419-1397-5_1, © Springer Science+Business Media, LLC 2010

injury was followed by a variety of reports of behavioral syndromes having similar characteristics that were linked to brain damage or dysfunction.

Alternative Terms for ADHD

Many different terms have been used to describe the hyperactive child with attention deficits and frequently associated learning disorders. Some have emphasized the symptoms (*hyperactivity, inattentiveness*), some refer to the presumed cause (*brain damage or dysfunction*), and others the educational problems (*perception and learning disorders*) associated with the behavior. The list of names for this syndrome is long, close to 40 in number, and the following are some examples:

- Hyperactive (hyperkinetic) child syndrome.
- Brain-injured child.
- Minimal brain dysfunction.
- Perceptually handicapped child.
- Deficits in attention, motor/perception (DAMP) (Landgren et al., 2000).

None of these terms is entirely satisfactory because the symptoms and causes of the syndrome are many and variable. Hyperactivity is the most common and striking complaint, but some children have normal or even lesser degrees of activity (*hypokinesis*), the syndrome expressed mainly by inattentiveness and distractibility. Subtle neurological abnormalities, perception deficits, and learning disabilities are frequently associated but not invariable findings. The current term ADHD emphasizes the symptoms but minimizes the importance of possible underlying causes and associated neurological and learning problems.

Evolution of Present Concept of ADHD

From the initial descriptions and concept of a brain damage syndrome, beginning with *postencephalitic behavior disorder*, in 1922, proceeding to the *brain-injured child* (1947) and the *perceptually handicapped child* (1963), and ending with *minimal brain dysfunction*, in 1966, the emphasis turned to symptoms, when the American Psychiatric Association included the syndrome in their Diagnostic and Statistical Manual (DSM) in 1968.

The first entry of the syndrome in DSM-II (1968) used the term *hyperkinetic reaction of childhood or adolescence.* In 1980, the DSM-III recognized two subtypes of a syndrome of *attention deficit disorder (ADD)* – *ADD with hyperactivity* and *ADD without hyperactivity.* In 1987, the DSM-III was revised (DSM-III-R) and the term *attention-deficit hyperactivity disorder (ADHD)* was used. Finally, in 1994, the DSM-IV now recognizes three subtypes of the syndrome: *ADHD-inattentive type*, *ADHD-hyperactive-impulsive type*, and *ADHD-combined type*. A minimum number of criteria are required for the diagnosis of each subtype.

Diagnostic Criteria for ADHD Subtypes

(1) *ADHD Inattentive* subtype, without hyperactivity (Code 314.00). At least six of the following nine symptoms have been noted for at least six months and are often present during school or play activities:

1. Makes careless mistakes;
2. Cannot maintain attention;
3. Does not listen when spoken to;
4. Fails to finish tasks;
5. Seems disorganized;
6. Avoids tasks;
7. Loses things;
8. Easily distracted;
9. Forgetful.

(2) *ADHD Hyperactive-Impulsive* subtype (Code 314.01). Six (or more) of the following symptoms have been present for at least six months: Hyperactivity:

1. Fidgety;
2. Leaves seat in classroom or at dinner table;
3. Runs or climbs excessively;
4. Cannot play quietly;
5. Always "on the go";
6. Talks a lot. Impulsivity:
7. Blurts out answers to questions;
8. Cannot wait in line or take turn;
9. Often interrupts.

(3) ADHD *Combined* type.

Criteria for both the *Inattentive* and the *Hyperactive-Impulsive* types have been present for at least 6 months.

The term *In Partial Remission* is applied to older children and adolescents whose symptoms have lessened with age or treatment and no longer add up to the required number for diagnosis.

Further Diagnostic Criteria

- The typical diagnostic symptoms of ADHD are a persistent pattern of inattention and/or hyperactivity and impulsiveness of an abnormal severity and frequency.

- Symptoms should have been present before the age of 7 years.
- Symptoms should be observed in at least two settings (school, home, workplace, or doctor's or psychologist's office).
- Symptoms are sufficient to impair academic, social, or occupational functions.
- Symptoms cannot be explained by a mental illness such as depression, anxiety, or personality disorder.

Questionnaires completed by parents, schoolteachers, psychologists, and physicians are used in arriving at the diagnosis. A neurological examination that uncovers signs of brain dysfunction or damage of a subtle type, and psychological tests showing deficits in perception and learning ability can be additional supportive evidence, although these findings are not essential for the diagnosis of ADHD. A specific chemical or laboratory test is not available, but abnormal levels of lead in the blood, thyroid hormone imbalance, or certain chromosomal anomalies (fragile X disease) may rarely provide an explanation for the symptoms.

ADHD, a Continuum or Medical Syndrome

In one large twin study reported from the Prince of Wales Hospital, Randwick, NSW, and involving almost 2000 families recruited from the Australian MRC Twin Registry, ADHD is viewed as a continuum and not a discrete medical syndrome. ADHD is explained as an inherited trait with liability and expression throughout the population, a deviance from an acceptable norm, and not restricted to an arbitrary number of symptoms or DSM diagnostic criteria. The need for treatment including medication is relative and dependent on multiple factors (Levy et al., 1997).

ADHD, a Medical Deficit or Social Deviance

Some skeptics argue that the symptoms of ADHD may be explained by a variation of "normal" behavior, a so-called boisterous child, or a reflection of our society. Sociologists criticize doctors for having "medicalized" symptoms that should be regarded as deviant behavior and an adaptation to the social environment (Conrad, 1973, Conrad and Schneider, 1980).

The medical concept of deviant behavior has humanitarian benefits for the individual, allowing less condemnation and less social stigma among peers and adults. The child with a diagnosis of ADHD is no longer the "bad boy" of the classroom. He has an "illness," requiring regular visits to the nurse for medicine at lunchtime. The disruptive and distractible behavior is not his fault. The diagnosis of ADHD is even used as an excuse for conduct disorders and drug addiction, sometimes exerting pressure on the justice system and claiming undeserved leniency.

The "medicalization" of ADHD, according to the sociologists, has followed the availability of a treatment, methylphenidate, to control the deviant behavior. They infer that the syndrome would not be recognized as an illness, if the paradoxical, quietening effect of stimulant medications had not been discovered (Bradley, 1937). By defining ADHD as a medical problem, we may be diverting attention from the family, school, or other factors in the social environment of probable underlying significance.

These arguments are an important reminder to physicians, parents, and teachers that the management of the child with ADHD must not rely exclusively on the prescription of stimulant or other medications. Treatment is "multimodal," including parental counseling, child behavior modification, and appropriate classroom size and teaching techniques, as well as medical intervention.

Prevalence of ADHD and Gender Factor

Approximately 5% of children and adolescents are affected, or at least one in every classroom. Boys are affected three to six times more commonly than girls. Some authorities have estimated the prevalence as high as 10%, and even 20%, in school children between 5 and 12 years of age. One report claimed a total of 3 million children with ADHD in the United States.

ADHD is recognized worldwide, but the reported prevalence varies in different countries, with less than 1 in a 1000 in a study of 10- and 11-year-old children in the Isle of Wight, UK (Rutter et al., 1970). The accuracy and comparison of these statistics are affected by the age of the study population, the variability of the patient selection, and the lack of agreement on the definition of diagnostic criteria.

In a study at Vanderbilt University, Nashville, TN, involving 8000 children in a Tennessee county, with ratings completed by 400 teachers, the estimates of prevalence of ADHD were higher when using the new diagnostic criteria listed in DSM-IV, as compared to DSM-III-R criteria (Wolraich et al., 1996). Prevalence rates were 7% for ADHD using DSM-III-R, and 11% with DSM-IV criteria, an increase of 57%. The inattentive (AD) subtype of ADHD occurred in 5%, the hyperactive-impulsive (H-I) type in 2.5%, and the combined type in 3.5%. Boys outnumbered girls with a 4:1 ratio for the ADHD-HI and 2:1 for ADHD-AD.

Age of Onset of ADHD

According to the DSM-IV criteria for diagnosis of ADHD, some symptoms should be present before the age of seven years. Hyperactivity is recognized most commonly at about four or five years of age, when the child starts school, although many parents complain about excessive motor restlessness in infancy In fact, some mothers have predicted the birth of a hyperactive child because of excessive fetal movements during pregnancy.

The environment will often influence the time of onset of symptoms. A child who is mildly restless at home or in the doctor's office may become hyperactive and distractible when entering a structured situation, such as a school classroom. On a one-to-one, student-teacher ratio, as in private tutoring, the child may function reasonably well, whereas in a large class of students, the symptoms of ADHD will immediately become apparent. Parents are sometimes dismayed at the reports from school, because in the home environment symptoms can be less obvious.

Summary

Attention deficit hyperactivity disorder (ADHD) is a neurobiological syndrome recognized under different terms for more than a century. Three subtypes of ADHD are described in the latest American Psychiatric Association Diagnostic Statistical Manual (DSM-IV): ADHD-inattentive type, ADHD-hyperactive-impulsive type, and ADHD-combined type. At least 6 of 9 listed symptoms present for at least 6 months are required in the diagnosis of each subtype. In addition, symptoms should be present before the age of 7 years and are not explained by mental illness, such as depression, anxiety, or personality disorder. ADHD is diagnosed in approximately 5% of children and adolescents, and boys are affected 3–6 times more often than girls.

References

Bradley C. The behavior of children receiving Benzedrine. *Am J Psychiatry*. 1937;94:577–585.
Conrad P. The discovery of hyperkinesis: notes on the medicalization of deviant behavior. *Soc Sci Med*. 1973;7:12–21.
Conrad P, Schneider JW. *Deviance and Medicalization. From Badness to Sickness*. St Louis, MO: CV Mosby; 1980.
Ebaugh F. Neuropsychiatric sequelae of acute epidemic encephalitis in children. *Am J Dis Child*. 1923;25:89–97.
English T. The after effects of head injuries. *Lancet*. 1904;1:485–489.
Hoffman H. Fidgety Philip. In: *The Oxford Dictionary of Quotations*. 2nd ed., London: Oxford University Press; 1955.
Hohman LB. Post-encephalitic behavior disorders in children. *Johns Hopkins HospBull*. 1922;380:372–375.
Kahn E, Cohen L. Organic drivenness: A brain stem syndrome and experience. *N Engl J Med*. 1934;210:748–756.
Landgren M, Kjellman B, Gillberg C. Deficits in attention, motor control and perception (DAMP): a simplified school entry examination. *Acta Paediatr*. 2000;89:302–309.
Leahly S, Sands I. Mental disturbances in children following epidemic encephalitis. *J Am Med Assoc*. 1921;76:373.
Levy F et al. ADHD as a continuum, not a discrete entity. *J Am Acad Child Adolesc Psychiatry*. 1997;36:737–744.

Psychiatric Association (APA). *Diagnostic American and Statistical Manual of Mental Disorders.* 4th ed, Washington, DC: APA; 1994.

Rutter M, Tizard J, Whitmore K.. *Education, Health and Behavior.* London: Longman; 1970.

Still GF. Some abnormal physical conditions in children. *Lancet.* 1902;1:1008–1012, 1077–1082, 1163–1168.

Strecker E, Ebaugh F. Neuropsychiatric sequelae of cerebral trauma in children. *Arch Neurol Psychiatry.* 1924;12:443–453.

Wolraich ML et al. Comparison of diagnostic criteria for attention-deficit hyperactivity disorder in a county-wide sample. *J Am Acad Child Adolesc Psychiatry.* 1996;35:319–324.

Chapter 2
Causative Factors

ADHD is a highly heritable disorder but in addition to genetic causes, acquired and environmental factors are sometimes uncovered that may be amenable to prevention or specific treatment. The causes of ADHD may be characterized as *idiopathic*, arising spontaneously from an unknown cause, *symptomatic* and secondary to a brain structural abnormality, or familial and presumed *genetic*. A majority of cases of ADHD are idiopathic or of uncertain cause. A delay in development or maturation of the nervous system is sometimes proposed as an explanation for ADHD, especially in children with mild or "soft" neurological deficits.

Etiological Classification

The etiologies of ADHD are sometimes classified by the time of their occurrence: (1) *prenatal*; (2) *perinatal*; and (3) *postnatal* (Table 2.1). The syndrome may be *genetic* and *familial*, or *acquired* and *environmental*. Rarely, a chromosomal anomaly is the underlying cause of ADHD.

Prenatal causes include developmental cerebral abnormality, maternal anemia, toxemia of pregnancy, alcohol and cocaine abuse, and tobacco smoke. Other environmental factors sometimes suspected are exposure to lead, PCBs and pesticides in the water and diet, lack of iodine and hypothyroidism. The season of birth may be a risk factor, and exposure to viral infections, especially influenza and viral exanthema, in the first trimester of pregnancy or at the time of birth has been correlated with the diagnosis of ADHD.

Perinatal etiological factors include the following: premature birth, breech delivery, anoxic-ischemic-encephalopathy, cerebral hemorrhage, meningitis, and encephalitis.

Postnatally, the infant may have suffered a head injury, meningitis, encephalitis, frequent attacks of otitis media, or low blood sugar. Drugs used to treat childhood illnesses, asthma and epilepsy, frequently cause or exacerbate hyperactive behavior and result in attention and learning deficits. The role of diet in the cause of ADHD is controversial, but the ingestion of food additives and sucrose, lack of omega 3 fatty acids, and allergies to certain foods are occasionally significant. A lack of iron

Table 2.1 Causes of ADHD

Time of effect	Causative factors
Prenatal	Cerebral maldevelopment, chromosome anomaly, infections, toxins, drugs, metabolic, endocrine disorder
Perinatal	Premature birth, encephalopathy, infection, hemorrhage
Postnatal	Infection, trauma, toxins, drugs, nutritional, endocrine disorder

Modified from Millichap (2008).

in the diet and anemia are documented potential causes and rarely, thyroid hormone dysfunction is associated with ADHD (Millichap, 2008). An abnormality in sensory input alleviated by oral potassium is proposed as a novel mechanism of ADHD in a 9-year-old boy with symptoms of sensory overstimulation and potassium sensitivity (Segal et al., 2007).

Evidence for a Neurological Basis for ADHD

The neurologic or anatomic theory of hyperactivity and ADHD is based on numerous experimental studies in animals, neurological and electroencephalographic (EEG) examinations, and magnetic resonance imaging (MRI) of the brain. Positron emission tomography (PET) studies, showing changes in glucose metabolism in the frontal lobes of the brain, point to a localized cerebral abnormality in adults who were hyperactive since childhood.

Neurological "soft" signs, including motor impersistence (an inability to maintain postures or movements), distractibility (an inability to maintain attention), and attentional control and response inhibition, are indicative of right-sided frontal cerebral lesions. Frontal cerebral lesions and their connections with the basal ganglia or striate cortex produce the greatest number and degree of hyperactive behavioral responses. The right prefrontal cortex has a role in attentional control and inhibiting responses, whereas the basal ganglia are involved in motor control and the execution of behavioral responses. Distractibility and impulsivity in ADHD children reflect deficits in response inhibition.

Injury or abnormal development of areas of the brain other than the frontal lobes may also be associated with the syndrome of ADHD and impairment of language and social skills. Cognitive dysfunction and ADHD are reported in children with temporal lobe lesions, and a connection with the fronto-striatal circuitry is possible in these cases.

At *Duke University Medical Center, Durham, NC,* deficits of cognitive function, language development, and social skills were reported in 4 children with bilateral medial temporal lobe (hippocampus) sclerosis, associated with severe epilepsy beginning in early childhood. MRI showed abnormal signals and 25% loss of hippocampal volume (DeLong and Heinz, 1997).

Temporal lobe arachnoid cyst is reported in association with ADHD in several childhood patients (Millichap, 1997). Although rare, the diagnosis of this association and syndrome points to the potential importance of prenatal factors in the cause of ADHD. The cause of arachnoid cyst is usually undetermined, but an injury to the fetal brain is likely, stemming from trauma, bleeding, or virus infection. In patients with increased intracranial pressure and complicating headaches or seizures, treatment sometimes requires surgery to drain the cyst, but generally the symptoms can be controlled by other more conservative measures.

MRI brain volume analyses. Measurements of various structures in the brain, using MRI quantitative techniques, have revealed changes in the development of the corpus callosum, a decreased volume of the right prefrontal cortex and basal ganglia, a smaller cerebellar vermis, and small cerebral volume. MRI measures of the right prefrontal cortex and basal ganglia correlate with response inhibition and task performance in ADHD children. Decreased cerebral volumes in some ADHD children may explain lower scores on IQ tests.

At the *Western Psychiatric Institute, University of Pittsburgh, PA,* MRI volumetric analyses in 26 children with ADHD compared to 26 normal controls showed correlations between task performance and prefrontal and caudate volume in the right hemisphere. Only right prefrontal measures correlated with performance of responses involving inhibition (Casey et al., 1997).

At the *National Institute of Mental Health, Bethesda, MD,* quantitative MRI studies in 46 right-handed boys with ADHD and 47 matched healthy controls found a smaller cerebellar vermis, especially involving the posterior inferior lobules, in the ADHD group. A cerebello-thalamo-prefrontal circuit dysfunction is postulated in ADHD (Berquin et al., 1998).

Localized cerebral hemisphere and cerebellar anomalies of development in ADHD are correlated with abnormal fronto-striatal-cerebellar function and sometimes with response to stimulant medication.

At the *University of California, Irvine,* volumetric MRI brain analyses in 15 male ADHD children compared to 15 normal controls showed smaller volumes of localized hemispheral structures. Smaller left basal ganglia (caudate nucleus specifically) was correlated with response to stimulant medication, whereas nonresponders had reversed caudate asymmetry (Filipek et al., 1997).

At the *University of Barcelona, Spain,* MRI measurements of the head of the caudate nucleus correlated with neuropsychological deficits and behavioral problems in 11 adolescents with ADHD. The ADHD group had a larger right caudate nucleus and a reversal of the normal L>R caudate asymmetry (Mataro et al., 1997).

The different anatomical sites of injury or lesion in the brain, sometimes detected in children with ADHD, can account for the varying symptoms and complications of the syndrome. The role of the right hemisphere and especially the right frontal lobe in the neurological basis for ADHD is stressed by Voeller (1990), my colleague, Charles Swisher (personal communication), and other neurologists, and is reviewed in "Progress in Pediatric Neurology I, II, & III" (Millichap, 1991, 1994, and 1997).

A frontal-motor cortex disconnection syndrome, or "lazy" frontal lobe, in ADHD is hypothesized on the basis of cerebral blood flow, EEG studies, and MRI volumetric analyses (Niedermeyer and Naidu, 1997). This concept is developed from the function of the frontal lobe as an inhibitor of excessive motor activity, children with

ADHD having disinhibited motor activity. The calming effect of methylphenidate may stem from a stimulatory effect on the frontal lobe causing motor inhibition.

EEG Abnormalities and ADHD. Epileptiform discharges in the EEG are reported in children with ADHD with varying frequencies, from 6% to as high as 53%. The indications for an EEG in ADHD include the following: (1) a history of seizures; (2) frequent "daydreaming"; (3) a history of head trauma, encephalitis or meningitis; and (4) as a precursor to treatment with stimulants in patients with a past or family history of epilepsy. A proportion of patients with ADHD have an increased susceptibility to seizures, based on EEG data.

Computerized power spectral analysis permitting statistical analysis of the EEG shows that boys, aged 9–12 years, with ADHD have increased theta (4.75 Hz) and decreased beta 1 (12.75–21 Hz) activity, when compared to controls matched for age and grade level (Mann, 1992). The increased theta is found in the frontal and central locations, and decreased beta in posterior and temporal locations.

EEG data from 184 boys with ADHD-combined type found three distinct EEG clusters or subtypes of children characterized by (a) increased slow wave activity and deficiencies of fast wave, (b) increased high amplitude theta with deficiencies of beta activity, and (c) an excess beta group (Clarke et al., 2001). Children with ADHD do not constitute a homogeneous group in EEG profile terms. Quantitative EEG data may provide more objective measurements of attentive difficulties in children with ADHD than are currently available from subjective questionnaires or rating scales. Variability of EEG characteristics must be recognized if the EEG is used as a reliable ADHD diagnostic tool sometime in the future.

Role of Genetic Factors in Etiology of ADHD

Parents will often admit that fathers and, less often, the mothers were hyperactive or had a learning problem during childhood. Occasionally, they will deny any childhood behavior or attention problem, despite their inability to sit quietly during the consultation. A history of siblings and cousins who have been diagnosed with ADHD and who have had a favorable response to stimulant medications is not uncommon.

The clear distinction between the effects of nature and nurture in the cause of ADHD is difficult to prove, and both genetic and acquired factors are important. In some patients, the cause may be purely inherited, in others, mainly acquired and environmental, and in many, a combination of both. Several methods are employed by epidemiologists to demonstrate the role of genetic factors as compared to environmental influences (Omen, 1973).

(1) ADHD prevalence in different geographic, ethnic, or racial populations.

In a study of 145 children diagnosed with ADHD at the Shaare Zedek Medical Center, Jerusalem, Israel, boys outnumbered girls by 3:1, 30% had siblings with learning disabilities compared to only 7% among control children without ADHD, and 34% were of North African descent, an ethnic background present in only 12%

of the population of Jerusalem. A familial-genetic factor in this group of patients was expressed by the preponderance of males, the increased frequency of learning disabilities in siblings, and an ethnic-related propensity to ADHD (Gross-Tsur et al., 1991).

(2) Risk of ADHD in first-degree relatives (parents, siblings, and children) of patients with ADHD compared to the general population.

Among 457 first degree relatives of children and adolescents referred to the Child Psychiatry Service, Massachusetts General Hospital, Boston, the risk of ADD, as well as antisocial and mood disorders, was significantly higher than among normal controls (Biederman et al., 1990).

(3) *Twin studies.* Identical, monozygotic (MZ) twins may be compared with fraternal, dizygotic (DZ) twins. If genetic factors are important, both MZ twins are affected (concordant), whereas concordance in DZ twins is lower and similar to that for ordinary siblings. DZ twins must be of the same sex in studies of ADHD, since there is a male preponderance. The extent to which MZ twins may be discordant (i.e. only one affected) is an indication of the influence of environmental factors in the cause of ADHD.

An evaluation of 10 pairs of twins, at least one having the hyperactive syndrome, showed that all four pairs of MZ twins were concordant, whereas only one of six DZ pairs was concordant. The MZ twins were all boys (Lopez, 1965). This study supports a genetic basis for ADHD.

The Minnesota Twin Family Study, involving 576 twin boys, aged 11 and 12, and analyses of teacher and maternal reports, confirmed the importance of genetic factors in the mediation of both inattention and hyperactivity-impulsivity subtypes of ADHD. Environmental factors had lesser contributions to the etiology of ADHD (Sherman et al., 1997).

At the *UCLA School of Medicine, Los Angeles, CA,* twin studies using interview assessment of ADHD showed 79% concordance in 37 monozygotic twins compared to 32% in 37 same sex dizygotic twins. ADHD is a familial disorder, with frequency five to sixfold greater among first-degree relatives than in the general population. Relatives of ADHD probands have increased rates of comorbid conditions, especially oppositional and conduct disorders, anxiety, mood disorders, and learning disabilities. Adoption studies support both a genetic basis for ADHD and environmental factors (Smalley, 1997).

(4) *Influence of environmental upbringing among MZ twins.* Comparison of MZ twins reared together versus MZ twins reared apart, in foster homes, allows epidemiologists to distinguish the influence of genetic from environmental factors within a family. Also, the incidence of ADHD in the biological vs the adoptive relatives or half-sibs can be determined.

In a study of full sibs and half-sibs of 14 children with minimal brain dysfunction (ADHD), all reared in foster homes, 50% of the full sibs vs 14% of the half-sibs had hyperactive behavior and attention deficits (Safer, 1969). These findings were more in favor of genetic than environmental influences in the cause of ADHD, although the study was flawed by a higher incidence of prematurity and neonatal difficulties among the full sibs, environmental factors known to cause ADHD.

Chromosomal Anomalies Associated with ADHD

Chromosomal syndromes are rare among ADHD-clinic patients. They include fragile X, velocardiofacial (22Q.11.2 deletion), Williams, Turner and Prader-Willi syndromes, and neurofibromatosis type 1 (Moore et al., 1996). In a study of 100 children (64 boys) with ADHD (combined type) and normal intelligence, 1 girl had a sex chromosome aneuploidy (47.XXX) and 1 boy had a permutation-sized allele for fragile X, but none showed the full mutation. Tests for 22q11.2 microdeletion were negative. In the absence of clinical signs or family history, routine chromosome analysis in children with ADHD is not generally recommended (Bastain et al., 2002).

Molecular Genetic Studies

The above reports point to the role of genetic factors in the cause of ADHD. The identification of a specific metabolic or enzyme marker is also required to prove an inherited predisposition. Studies focused on catecholaminergic candidates support the involvement of the dopamine receptor and dopamine transporter genes (DAT1). Deficits in dopamine-modulated frontal-striatal circuits are correlated with subtypes of ADHD. The relation of dopamine deficits to fetal and perinatal stresses may explain the mechanism of environmental etiologies of ADHD (Swanson et al., 2007). Preterm birth complicated by susceptibility to cerebral ischemia may contribute to increased dopamine receptor availability, deficient dopaminergic transmission, and subsequent development of ADHD (Lou et al., 2004).

Evidence of environmental mediators in ADHD has been demonstrated in twin studies. Affected twins have greater exposure to risk factors such as maternal smoking, lower birth weights, and delayed growth and development compared with unaffected co-twins (Lehn et al., 2007). Gene-environment interaction is increasingly recognized as an important mechanism in the etiology and development of ADHD, with some genes (e.g. DAT1) affecting the individual sensitivity to environmental etiological factors (Thapar et al., 2007).

Environmental Factors in Etiology

The evidence for environmental and acquired factors, although often presumptive, is perhaps stronger than the genetic data in the search for causes of ADHD (Millichap, 2008). *Pregnancy- and birth-related risk factors* include maternal smoking and nicotine, exanthema, maternal anemia, breech delivery, prematurity, low birth weight, hypoxic-ischemic-encephalopathy, small head circumference, cocaine and alcohol exposure, and iodine and thyroid deficiency. *Childhood illnesses* linked to ADHD include viral infections, meningitis, encephalitis, otitis media, anemia, cardiac disease, thyroid disease, epilepsy, and autoimmune and metabolic disorders. Head injury involving the frontal lobes, toxins and drugs, and nutritional disorders are additional risk factors. The relation of dietary factors to ADHD is often controversial, especially food additives, food allergies, sucrose, gluten sensitivity, and fatty acid and iron deficiency. Of all the environmental factors implicated, maternal smoking and nicotine exposure attract the most attention in the literature, but in practice, cigarette smoking is almost invariably denied.

Role of Adverse Home and School Environments

Adverse home environments and overcrowded classrooms may contribute to and exacerbate hyperactivity and inattentiveness in a child with ADHD. However, these factors alone are rarely the explanation, and intrinsic genetic or acquired causes must always be investigated.

The influence of parents with psychiatric illness on the functioning of children with ADHD and normal control children was studied at the Pediatric Psychopharmacology Unit in Psychiatry, *Massachusetts General Hospital, Boston, MA*. The frequency of adverse family environments, including chronic family conflict, poor family union, and mothers with psychiatric problems, was greater among 140 ADHD compared to 120 normal children (Biederman et al., 1995).

Early recognition of these environmental factors should lead to prompt intervention and improved outcome.

In a study of psychiatric disorders in families of children with ADHD, at the Department of Pediatrics, *Wyler and La Rabida Children's Hospitals, University of Chicago,* alcoholism, drug abuse, depression, learning disabilities, and/or ADHD were more common among parents of ADHD than control children (with Down syndrome) (Roizen et al., 1996).

Children with a family history of psychiatric disorders should be screened for ADHD.

ADHD in Adopted Children

In a previous analysis of the author's patients, the incidence of adoption among children with the hyperactive syndrome was 12% and more than three times the national incidence of adoption in that year (Millichap, 1975). A 17% rate of adoption was reported in another study of ADD children, 8 times that found in a normal control group or in the general population (Deutch et al., 1982). Behavioral and psychiatric problems are not increased in the foster families of hyperactive adoptive children, according to another study (Morrison and Stewart, 1973).

Although it is generally believed that behavior problems are more prevalent among adopted children, the occurrence of adverse psychological environments in foster or adoptive placements must not be assumed. An increased likelihood of insults to the fetus or newborn baby during unwanted pregnancies and births and possible genetic anomalies are more plausible explanations. In the author's ADD clinic at *Children's Memorial Hospital, Chicago*, cocaine exposure during pregnancy and birth is frequently reported by adoptive parents of foster children but is only rarely admitted by a biological parent.

Biochemical Basis for ADHD

Evidence is accumulating that changes in the brain chemistry – the catecholamine *neurotransmitters* (dopamine, norepinephrine, and serotonin) – might account for hyperactivity, inattentiveness, and other symptoms of ADHD. The central nervous system stimulants, dextroamphetamine and methylphenidate (*Ritalin*®), benefit ADHD by increasing catecholamine concentrations in the brain. Catecholamine metabolism and levels of norepinephrine are related to arousal, attention span, and motor activity.

The biochemical studies in children with ADHD are experimental. Measurements of metabolites, or breakdown products, of dopamine and norepinephrine in the urine or of enzymes in the blood are not of practical significance in the diagnosis and treatment of ADHD, but they increase our understanding of the neurobiology of ADHD (Yehuda, 1986; Zametkin and Rapoport, 1987).

Infectious Causes of ADHD

Viral infections during pregnancy, at birth, and in early childhood are linked to an increased risk of ADHD. In a case-controlled study in Italy, the frequency of measles, varicella, or rubella, in mothers of children who developed ADHD is significantly higher than in controls (Arpino et al., 2005). Other viral infections associated with an increased prevalence of ADHD and learning disorders include HIV, enterovirus 71, and varicella zoster encephalitis. Febrile seizures, frequently associated with human herpesvirus 6 infection in the United States and with influenza A in Asia, are a risk factor for development of ADHD (Millichap, 2008). A possible relation between ADHD and streptococcal infection and a causative role for otitis media require confirmation.

Perinatal and Early-Life Risk Factors

Various centers internationally have reviewed the roles of premature birth and perinatal hypoxic-ischemic encephalopathy in the pathophysiology of ADHD. At the *John F Kennedy Institute, Glostrup, Denmark*, up to one-third of premature infants with birth weights of <1500 g have ADHD by 5–7 years of age (Lou, 1996). Birth histories of 196 children with ADHD followed in Iceland showed a statistically significant increased risk associated with low birth weight, young maternal age, and cesarean delivery (Valdimarsdottir et al., 2006). Advances in NICU nursing care and improved survival rates among premature infants have lead to an increase in the importance of perinatal risk factors for ADHD. In contrast, a case-control study at the *Mayo Clinic* found that pregnancy and labor, low birth weight, and twin birth were not correlated with ADHD, while male gender and low parental education levels were positive risk factors (St Sauver et al., 2004).

Postnatal Risk Factors

Cerebral trauma, meningitis, encephalitis, metabolic and endocrine disorders, especially thyroid dysfunction, toxins and drugs, and nutritional deficiencies, additives, and food sensitivities are factors known to be associated with ADHD. A genetic factor and inherited predisposition are likely basic causes, and environmental factors are probably secondary, acting as a trigger. Some potentially preventable ADHD environmental causes include hypoglycemia, iron, zinc, and iodine deficiencies.

Head Injury as a Cause of ADHD and Learning Disorders

Head injury, even mild in degree, in young children warrants observation and follow-up for possible behavior and cognitive impairments. Hyperactive behavior was directly correlated with the severity of head injury in a study of 95 children, aged 5–15 years, followed at the *Johns Hopkins University, Baltimore* (Greenspan and MacKenzie, 1994). The risk of functional limitations following injury was increased in children with previous chronic health problems and those who sustained lower extremity injuries in addition to head injury.

Mild head injury, not sufficient to require admission to hospital for observation, can result in learning deficits and impairment of reading and school performance in young children. Compared to a control group of preschool children with minor injury not involving the head, 78 head-injured preschoolers tested at one year after injury had visual perception problems and an increased incidence of dyslexia (Wrightson et al., 1995). The development of visual skills necessary for reading was interrupted by the mild head injury.

Math and spelling abilities were impaired in a 17-year-old boy who had sustained a right hemisphere injury in infancy. Investigations using a functional MRI at the *University of Maryland, Baltimore*, showed activation of the left hemisphere while the patient performed arithmetic calculations. Visuospatial skills normally subserved by the right hemisphere had been transferred to the left hemisphere after the injury, causing a "crowding effect" and disproportionate impairment of math and reading skills in comparison to language development (Levin et al., 1996).

At *Columbia University and New York State Psychiatric Institute*, low-birth-weight children, with neonatal cranial ultrasound abnormalities suggestive of white matter injury, were at increased risk for neuropsychiatric disorders, especially ADHD, by the age of 6 years (Whitaker et al., 1997).

Brain injury at an early age can lead to reorganization of the locations in the brain where attention, language, and cognitive function are represented.

Hypoglycemia and ADHD

Hypoglycemia in a newborn infant, if unrecognized and untreated, can cause convulsions and brain damage that later may result in mental retardation or learning disorders and ADHD. Transient hypoglycemia may occur in infants with birth anoxia or other forms of perinatal stress or in neonates born to mothers with diabetes or toxemia.

Early onset childhood diabetes, before the age of 5 years, is often complicated by episodes of severe hypoglycemia that result in mild cognitive dysfunction, whereas late-onset diabetes, after the age of 5 years, and occasional episodes of severe hypoglycemia have no effect on cognitive function, according to a study in 28 diabetic children at the *Trondheim University Hospital, Norway* (Bjorgaas et al., 1997).

Transient reactive hypoglycemia, following a diet of high sugar content, may be associated with behavioral symptoms seen with ADHD. A rapid rise in blood glucose can result in a heightened insulin secretion, with resultant hypoglycemic symptoms.

Role of Sugar and Other Dietary Factors in ADHD

Parents frequently note a worsening of hyperactivity and distractibility after the child with ADHD has eaten a high carbohydrate meal or a lot of candy. While the majority of scientifically controlled studies have failed to demonstrate a significant adverse effect, isolated reports tend to support the parents' observations.

In a study at *Yale University School of Medicine, New Haven, CT,* a fall in blood glucose at 3–5 h after a glucose drink was accompanied by symptoms of hypoglycemia (shakiness, sweating, weakness, and tachycardia) in children but not in adults. The reactive lowering of the blood glucose had stimulated a rise in plasma epinephrine, twice as high in children as in adults, sufficient to induce the symptoms of hypoglycemia. A measure of cognitive function, using evoked potentials, was significantly reduced when blood glucose was lowered below 75 mg/dl in children, but was preserved in adults until the level fell to 54 mg/dl (Jones et al., 1995).

Children appear to be more vulnerable to the effects of hypoglycemia on cognitive function than are adults. A diagnosis of excess sugar ingestion and reactive hypoglycemia as a cause of ADHD may be entertained when the child also suffers from more characteristic symptoms, including nervousness, tremor, sweating, dizziness, or palpitations.

At the *Child Psychiatry Branch and Laboratory of Developmental Psychology, NIMH, Bethesda, MD,* the effects of glucose, sucrose, saccharin, and aspartame on aggression and motor activity in 30 boys, aged 2–6 years, were compared. Eighteen boys were classed as "sugar responders" on parent questionnaires and 12 were "non-responders." Single dose challenges with sugar or sweetener, in a randomized, double-blind study, produced no significant differences in aggression or activity levels, as measured by teacher and parent ratings. The base-line duration of aggression in the alleged sugar responders correlated with the daily total sugar consumption, but acute sugar loading did not increase aggression or activity in preschool children (Krnesi et al., 1987).

At the *Schneider Children's Hospital, New York,* the effect of a sucrose challenge on aggressive behavior and attention was studied in a sample of hyperactive boys with ADD and age-matched control subjects (Wender and Solanto, 1991). Aggression was not modified, but inattention measured by a continuous performance task was increased following sugar ingestion in the ADHD group. Conners CK at the *National Children's Hospital, Washington, DC,* reports that behavioral effects of sugar in children with ADHD may be demonstrated if the sucrose challenge follows a high carbohydrate breakfast. The effects are reversed or blocked if the child has a protein meal before or with the ingestion of sugar (Yehuda, 1987)

An analysis of 16 published studies on the effects of sucrose on behavior and cognition of children with ADHD, conducted at *Vanderbilt University, Nashville, TN,* failed to demonstrate a significant adverse effect in the group as a whole, but a small effect in some sets of ADHD children could not be ruled out (Wolraich et al., 1995). Aspartame (Nutrasweet®) used as a control in these studies was considered to have no adverse effect on behavior or cognition (Shaywitz et al., 1994), but further investigation of the safety of aspartame may be indicated. Some authorities have demonstrated an exacerbation of EEG seizure discharges and of migraine headaches following aspartame ingestion.

Feingold Theory of Food Additives as a Cause of ADHD

Controlled studies of the additive-free, Feingold diet have failed to demonstrate a significant benefit in children with ADHD, except in an occasional pre-school child. However, some parents still believe that their children are reactive to foods containing artificial coloring, flavoring agents, and preservatives. They avoid apples, luncheon meats, sausage, hot dogs, gum, candies, cake mixes, oleomargarine, and ice cream. Flavored cold drinks, soda pop, and medicines containing aspirin are also excluded from the Feingold diet (1975).

The evidence for and against the Feingold theory is reviewed in Chap. 10. Scientific panels, established to study the efficacy of the diet and sponsored by the FDA, criticized the treatment and theory for lack of controls and statistical validity. Numerous studies of the effects of food additives on behavior followed, including additive-containing challenges. Small subgroups of younger children were found to react adversely to color additives in short-term trials, but the overwhelming benefits claimed for the Feingold diet were not substantiated (National Institutes of Health Consensus Panel, 1982).

The proof of food additive toxicity and relation to hyperactive behavior is difficult to determine. Questionnaires completed by parents, teachers, and psychologists may be biased, for or against, and may not address behavioral symptoms susceptible to the additive-free diet. Interest in the Feingold hypothesis and dietary treatment of ADHD has waned in the United States but waxes in Europe and Australia, where research continues on the use of elimination and hypoallergenic diets for the treatment of a variety of childhood neurobehavioral disorders.

Irritability, restlessness, and sleep disturbance rather than attention deficit were the behavioral patterns associated with the ingestion of azo dye food colorings (tartrazine and carmoisine) in a small, double-blind controlled study at the *Royal Children's Hospital, Victoria, Australia* (Rowe, 1988). The author concluded that behavioral rating questionnaires not including sleep habits may fail to identify specific reactors to food additives.

Role of Food Allergy in ADHD

Food allergy is proposed as a possible factor in the cause of ADHD. Chocolate, cow milk, egg, citrus, wheat, nuts, and cheese have triggered hyperactive behavior in some susceptible patients. A hyposensitization treatment with intradermal injections of food allergens (EPD) in 40 children with ADHD was conducted at the *Universitatskinderklinik, Munchen, Germany*, and the *Great Ormond Street Hospital, London* (Egger et al., 1992). Of 20 children receiving the EPD injections, 16 no longer reacted toward hyperactivity-provoking foods, compared to 4 of 20 who received placebo shots. A hypoallergenic, elimination diet has been used occasionally in practice, with variable results (Millichap, 1986). The role of food hypersensitivity as a cause of ADHD is difficult to document, the cooperation of neurologist, allergist, and dietician being essential. The hypoallergenic diet deserves further study.

Iron Deficiency and ADHD

Researchers in Paris, France report evidence of iron deficiency in children with ADHD. Serum ferritin levels were <30 ng/ml in 84% of children with ADHD vs 18% of control non-ADHD children; 32% had levels of <15 ng/ml vs 3% of controls. The authors report improvements in attention and behavior following supplemental iron (Konofal et al., 2004).

In contrast, our experience in Chicago shows that a mean serum ferritin level of 39.9 ± 40.6 ng/ml in ADHD children is not different than that of control children with no ADHD, but 18% of children with ADHD have levels below 20 ng/ml that are considered abnormal. None had evidence of iron-deficiency anemia.

A comparison of clinical characteristics of children with the lowest serum ferritin levels (< 20 ng/ml) and those with highest serum ferritin levels (> 60 ng/ml) show no significant difference in severity or frequency of ADHD and comorbid symptoms or response to medications (Millichap et al., 2006). An uncontrolled trial of iron supplement was ineffective and did not provide a substitute for medication in the management of ADHD. A causative role for low serum ferritin levels in ADHD was not confirmed in our patient cohort. Differences in mean iron storage levels in the French and Chicago-based studies may explain the variation in response to iron supplements. Further controlled trials of iron supplements may be indicated. Routine serum ferritin levels in children with ADHD may be justified.

Role of Zinc in ADHD

Several controlled studies, mainly in Turkey and Iran, countries with suspected endemic zinc deficiency, demonstrate a deficiency of zinc in patients with ADHD and a beneficial response to zinc sulfate supplements (Arnold et al., 2005). In another study, low serum zinc levels were correlated with inattention but not with hyperactivity/impulsivity (Arnold and DiSilvestro, 2005). Some researchers recommend zinc sulfate supplements as adjunctive therapy with methylphenidate. In the United States, routine serum zinc levels in children presenting with ADHD are probably not warranted.

Iodine Deficiency, Thyroid Function and ADHD

Iodine deficiency and hypothyroidism are prenatal and postnatal risk factors for ADHD in some environments. Optimal iodine intake is essential for normal thyroid function and the prevention of learning disabilities and academic underachievement. In the United States, iodine is present in the diet in adequate amounts but in underdeveloped countries, iodine deficiency is a common occurrence. Estimates find 200 million people affected by iodine deficiency diseases and 800 million at risk worldwide, a total of 1 billion at risk of brain maldevelopment or malfunction. A prospective study of the neuropsychological development of offspring of women from an iodine-deficient area in Italy found ADHD in 69%; no cases of ADHD were reported in an iodine sufficient area. The mothers were hypothyroxinemic at early gestation, resulting in reduction of triiodothyronine available to the developing fetal brain (Vermiglio et al., 2004). Endemic cretinism (congenital hypothyroidism) is the most serious complication of iodine deficiency. Milder forms of iodine deficiency can result in impaired cognitive function and learning disabilities in later childhood. Iodine deficiency, a major international public health problem especially affecting underdeveloped countries, may be prevented by iodinized salt in the diet.

At the *University of Groningen, The Netherlands,* continuous performance tasks, measures of the ability to sustain attention, were used to study 48 children with early treated congenital hypothyroidism and 35 healthy controls. Impairments of sustained attention were correlated with low pre-treatment thyroid hormone levels but not with onset of treatment for hypothyroidism. Declines in sustained-attention task performance were related to cognitive, motor, and motivational deficits (Kooistra et al., 1996).

At the *Sanjay Gandhi Postgraduate Institute of Medical Sciences, Lucknow, India,* 100 boys with prolonged iodine deficiency, not suffering from cretinism and selected for their ability to read and write, were slow learners and had impaired motivation to achieve (Tiwari et al., 1996).

Iodine deficiency not resulting in cretinism can cause learning disabilities and poor academic motivation.

Thyroid dysfunction. Impairments of cognition, attention, and behavior may occur with hypo- or hyper-thyroidism. Case reports of thyrotoxicosis and ADHD are rare, and symptoms may be subtle, leading to a missed diagnosis. In 3 patients with no characteristic signs of hyperthyroidism, treatment resulted in control of hyperactivity, increased attention span, and improved language function (Suresh et al., 1999). The authors recommend routine thyroid screening in children with ADHD. In the neurology ADHD clinic at *Children's Memorial Hospital, Chicago,* using routine thyroid screening we have encountered four cases of hyperthyroidism in one year, two with goiter.

ADHD is reported in patients with generalized resistance to thyroid hormone (GRTH), a disease caused by mutations in the thyroid receptor B gene. GRTH is characterized by reduced responsiveness of peripheral and pituitary tissues to thyroid hormone. In families with a history of GRTH studied at the *National Institutes of Health, Bethesda, MD,* 70% of affected children met the criteria for ADHD (Hauser et al., 1993). In another study, the prevalence of ADHD in patients with GRTH was 46% (Weiss et al., 1993). Despite some reports of a lack of association between GRTH and ADHD (Elia et al., 1994), screening of patients with a family history of thyroid dysfunction is recommended.

Lead Exposure as a Cause of ADHD

Clinical reports suggest that lead-exposed children may be distractible and hyperactive, but few studies have examined the effects of lead on behavior using statistical controls. A characteristic "behavioral signature" associated with lead exposure has not been identified (Bellinger, 1995). Proof of cause and effect is often lacking, especially for conditions such as pervasive development disorder and speech articulation problems.

Although the research is controversial, cognitive deficits have been correlated with blood lead levels of 10 mcg/dl or higher. Questions regarding risk of lead exposure at home, the school, or playground are important in children presenting with learning and behavior disorders. Preschool blood lead determinations are mandatory in some communities, but testing is appropriate in children diagnosed with ADHD and living in high-risk environments.

At the *Department of Community Medicine, University of Adelaide, Australia,* a study of low level lead exposure and effects on intelligence, which began in 1979, has been followed into the primary school age range. In 494 children, aged 7 years, from a lead smelting community, the IQ was inversely related to antenatal and post-natal blood lead concentrations, even at 10 mcg/dl levels. An increase in blood lead from 10 to 30 mcg/dl caused deficits in verbal IQ and full scale IQ of 6 and 5 points, respectively (Baghurst et al., 1992).

Three longitudinal studies in different locations (Australia, Boston, and Cincinnati) have demonstrated that lead-associated decreased intelligence is persistent across cultures, racial and ethnic groups, and social and economic classes. The finding is not limited to socially and economically disadvantaged children (Mahaffey, 1992).

Cocaine-Exposed Infants at Risk of ADHD

Cocaine-exposed infants require careful follow-up for early diagnosis and therapy of neurobehavioral complications. A history of prenatal cocaine exposure is common in foster children with ADHD attending our ADD clinic. A cause and effect is presumed but not proven.

At the *University of Miami School of Medicine, FL,* a study of 30 preterm cocaine-exposed infants compared to normal controls found smaller head circumference at birth, and a higher incidence of cerebral hemorrhage, restless sleep, agitated behavior, and tremulousness (Scafidi et al., 1996). The signs of abnormal brain development and excitation in cocaine-exposed infants were associated with higher levels of norepinephrine and dopamine in the urine, neurotransmitter chemicals important in the mechanism of ADHD. Hormonal changes, with higher cortisol levels and lower plasma insulin levels, were also reported in the cocaine-exposed newborns.

At the *University of Florida, Gainesville, FL,* cranial ultrasound examinations of 134 cocaine-exposed compared to 132 control newborns found an increased incidence of brain cysts and enlarged ventricles, possibly related to cocaine effects on brain development (Behnke et al., 1998).

At the *Women and Infants Hospital, Brown University School of Medicine, Providence, RI,* increased muscle tone and motor activity, jerky movements, startles, tremors, and back arching were observed in 20 infants with prenatal exposure to cocaine, alcohol, marijuana, and nicotine cigarettes (Napiorkowski et al., 1996). Signs of brain excitability were related only to cocaine and were neither apparent in the 17 infants exposed to alcohol, marijuana, and nicotine without cocaine, nor in the 20 drug-free infants.

At the *Children's Hospital, Boston, MA,* dose-related effects of cocaine on neurobehavior were demonstrated in exposed infants examined at 3 weeks of age. Heavily exposed infants showed impaired regulation of arousal and greater excitability than lightly or unexposed infants (Tronick et al., 1996).

Effects of prenatal cocaine on behavior and development noted in infancy are likely precursors of ADHD in later childhood. A combination of cocaine exposure and poor nutrition is a cumulative risk factor for impaired infantile motor performance and later cognitive development in inner-city minority infants.

Fetal Exposure to Alcohol, Marijuana, or Cigarettes and Increased Risk of ADHD

Behavioral problems are one of the characteristics of the "fetal alcohol syndrome" (FAS). Alcohol use during pregnancy and breast-feeding may cause delay in an infant's development and even an increased risk of brain hemorrhage (Holzman et al., 1995).

In a study of 64 alcoholic families at the *Karolinska Institute, Stockholm, Sweden*, children were retarded in development and had more behavioral problems than controls up to 4 years of age. Boys were more vulnerable than girls. Behavioral disorders were more pronounced when both parents were alcoholic (Nordberg et al., 1994).

At *Sahlgren University Hospital, Goteborg, Sweden,* 26 children of mothers who abused alcohol during pregnancies were followed throughout childhood and were examined at 11–14 years of age for neuropsychiatric, psychological, and social problems. Of 24 children seen at follow-up, 10 had ADHD, 2 had Asperger syndrome, and one had mild mental retardation and autistic spectrum disorder. The severity of the disorder was correlated with the degree of alcohol exposure in utero. Children whose mothers discontinued alcohol consumption by the 12th week of gestation developed normally and had no learning problems in school (Aronson et al., 1997). Biological, not psychosocial, factors are responsible for ADHD in children with fetal alcohol syndrome.

Maternal tobacco or marijuana smoking. A systematic search of the literature found 24 studies concerning maternal tobacco smoking published between 1973 and 2002. All reports indicated an increased risk of ADHD in the offspring (Linnet et al., 2003). Maternal cigarette smoking has been linked to impairments of cognitive function and memory, academic under-achievement, and behavioral problems in children exposed during pregnancy (Drews et al., 1996).

In a follow-up study of 6-year old children studied at *Carleton University, Ottawa, Ontario, Canada*, prenatal marijuana was associated with errors of omission in tasks of vigilance, reflecting a deficit in sustained attention (Fried et al., 1992). Cigarette smoking, marijuana use, and alcohol excess during pregnancy may have adverse effects on the behavior and attention of the infant and child, but a definite causative role in ADHD has not been established.

PCBs and Other Environmental Toxins as Potential Causes of ADHD

Environmental contaminants of our food and water supplies include PCBs (polychlorinated biphenyls), PBBs (polybrominated biphenyls), nitrates, DDT, dioxin, mercury, and lead. DDT and other pesticides, including dioxin, and PCBs have not been produced since the 1970s. Despite the ban on the manufacture of these chemicals, dangerous concentrations persist in the water of rivers and inland lakes.

PCBs were dumped years ago as waste products from electrical transformer, capacitor, and plasticizer factories. From the sediment at the bottom of harbors, hazardous waste residues pollute the water and are eaten by microscopic organisms and fish. From fish the chemicals are passed to birds and humans, causing various ailments including cancer and reproductive problems (Millichap, 1993, 1995). Man is the final consumer in the food chains, and he is exposed to the greatest concentrations of any environmental poison.

While regulatory control measures have substantially reduced the PCB contamination of animal feeds and food products by spillage, those subgroups of the population who regularly consume fish caught in lakes and streams are still at risk of poisoning. Surveys and analyses of fish from the Hudson River in New York State and from Lake Michigan showed significant levels of contamination with PCBs in excess of 5 ppm.

Studies designed to assess the health hazard of PCB exposure from Lake Michigan fish showed a correlation between the quantity of fish consumed and the concentration of PCB in blood and breast milk of participants in the studies. Those eating higher amounts of fish had significantly higher blood levels of PCB. Children born to women who routinely consumed Lake Michigan sport fish displayed impaired short-term memory function on both verbal and quantitative tests. In a study at *Wayne State University, Detroit, MI*, cognitive function was tested at 11 years of age in 212 children exposed prenatally to PCBs (Jacobson and Jacobson, 1996). Long-term intellectual impairment affected memory, attention, and reading ability, deficits frequently found in children with ADHD.

Developmental neurotoxicity of PCBs is reviewed in a publication from the *Institute of Environmental Studies, University of Illinois at Urbana-Champaign, Illinois* (Schantz, 1996). Studies included reports from Yusho, Japan; Yucheng, Taiwan; Michigan; North Carolina; Oswego, NY; New Bedford, MA; on Inuit people in the Arctic regions of Quebec; and in Faroe Islanders. Methylmercury poisoning could be an additional contaminant in some studies. Children born to mothers exposed to PCBs showed abnormalities in behavior and development, including higher activity levels, lower IQ scores, decreased birth weight and head circumference, deficits in memory at 4 years, and delays in psychomotor development. The public health implications of low-level PCB exposure were compared to those of lead exposure. The effect of PCB was either by direct injury to the brain in the prenatal period or secondary to effects on thyroid function.

At *Odense University, Denmark,* a study of 1022 children born in 1986–1987 in the Faroe Islands to mothers who had consumed methylmercury-polluted pilot whale meat found deficits in language, attention, and memory at 7 years of age (Grandjean et al., 1997).

Subtle alterations in neuropsychological functioning caused by exposure to these environmental toxins are proposed as potential causes for some cases of ADHD and learning disabilities.

Role of Diet During Infancy in the Cause of ADHD

Diets during infancy have been studied in relation to adult diseases such as hypertension and heart attack. Researchers at *Columbia University, New York*, have studied the rate of weight gain and diet-dependent changes in biochemistry, physiology, and behavior of 142 preterm infants fed varied protein and energy intakes (de Klerk et al., 1997). Rapidly growing infants had increased heart rates, respiratory rates, active sleep time, and decreased EEG frequencies compared to slow growing infants. Shifts in the balance of catecholamine and serotonergic neurotransmitters, similar to those reported with ADHD, were proposed as the cause of the changes in autonomic responses related to diet and rapid growth. Nutrition and weight gain during infancy may be a factor in the etiology of ADHD.

Summary

The cause of ADHD is frequently unknown or *idiopathic* but in some cases, *symptomatic* and secondary to a brain structural abnormality, traumatic or encephalitic. A familial, genetic factor in an estimated 80% of cases may involve the dopamine receptor and transporter genes, but gene-environment interaction is recognized as the important mechanism in the etiology of ADHD. Environmental factors may occur prenatally, in the perinatal period, or postnatally. They include developmental cerebral abnormalities, infections, toxins, premature birth, encephalopathy, and nutritional and endocrine disorders. A neuroanatomical theory for the symptoms of ADHD is based on the clinical examination and neurological "soft signs," electroencephalographic abnormalities, magnetic resonance imaging and brain volume studies, and positron emission tomography. Numerous experimental studies in animals have demonstrated hyperactive behavior elicited by prefrontal cerebral lesions. Head injury, even mild in degree, in young children is correlated with learning and behavior disorders. A neurochemical basis for ADHD is also proposed involving catecholamine neurotransmitters, a theory supported by the beneficial effects of stimulant medications.

The recognition of environmental factors in the etiology of ADHD should lead to prompt intervention, improved outcome, and in some cases, prevention of ADHD.

References

Arnold LE, Bozzolo H, Hollway J, et al. Serum zinc correlates with parent- and teacher-rated inattention in children with attention-deficit/hyperactivity disorder. *J Child Adolesc Psychopharmacol.* 2005;15:628–636.

Arnold LE, DiSilvestro RA. Zinc in attention-deficit/hyperactivity disorder. *J Child Adolesc Psychopharmacol.* 2005;15:619–627.

Aronson M et al. Attention deficits and autistic spectrum problems in children exposed to alcohol during gestation: a follow-up study. *Dev Med Child Neurol.* 1997;39:583–587.

Arpino C, Marzio M, D'Argenzio L, Longo B, Curatolo P. Exanthematic diseases during pregnancy and attention-deficit/hyperactivity disorder (ADHD). *Eur J Pediatr Neurol.* 2005;9: 363–365.

Baghurst PA et al. Environmental exposure to lead and children's intelligence at the age of seven years. *N Engl J Med.* 1992;327:1279–1284.

Bastain TM, Lewczyk CM, Sharp WS, et al. Cytogenetic abnormalities in attention-deficit/hyperactivity disorder. *J Am Acad Child Adolesc Psychiatry.* 2002;41:806–810.

Behnke M et al. Fetal cocaine exposure and brain abnormalities. *J Pediatr.* 1998;132:291–294.

Bellinger DC. Interpreting the literature on lead and child development: the neglected role of the "experimental system". *Neurotoxicol Teratol.* 1995;17:201–212.

Berquin PC et al. Cerebellum in attention-deficit hyperactivity disorder. A morphometric MRI study. *Neurology.* 1998;50:1087–1093.

Biederman J et al. Family-genetic and psychosocial risk factors in DSM-III attention deficit disorder. *J Am Acad Child Adolesc Psychiatry.* 1990;29:527–533.

Biederman J et al. Impact of adversity on functioning and comorbidity in children with attention-deficit hyperactivity disorder. *J Am Acad Child Adolesc Psychiatry.* 1995;34:1495–1503.

Bjorgaas M et al. Cognitive function in type 1 diabetic children with and without episodes of severe hypoglycemia. *Acta Paediatr.* 1997;86:148–153.

Casey BJ et al. Implication of right frontostriatal circuitry in response inhibition and attention-deficit/hyperactivity disorder. *J Am Acad Child Adolesc Psychiatry.* 1997;36:374–383.

Clarke AR, Barry RJ, McCarthy R, Selikowitz M. EEG-defined subtypes of children with attention-deficit/hyperactivity disorder. *Clin Neurophysiol.* 2001;112:2098–2105.

de Klerk A et al. Diet and infant behavior. *Acta Paediatr.* 1997;86(Suppl 422):65–68.

DeLong GR, Heinz ER. The clinical syndrome of early-life bilateral hippocampal sclerosis. *Ann Neurol.* 1997;42:11–17.

Deutch C et al. Overrepresentation of adoptees in children with attention deficit disorder. *Behav Genet.* 1982;12:231–237.

Drews CD et al. Maternal smoking is a preventable cause of mental retardation. *Pediatrics.* 1996;97:547–553.

Egger J et al. Controlled trial of hyposensitization in children with food-induced hyperkinetic syndrome. *Lancet.* 1992;339:1150–1153.

Elia J, Rapoport JL et al. Thyroid function and attention-deficit hyperactivity disorder. *J Am Acad Child Adolesc Psychiatry.* 1994;33:169–172.

Feingold BF. *Why Your Child Is Hyperactive.* New York: Random House; 1975.

Filipek PA et al. Volumetric MRI analysis comparing subjects having attention-deficit hyperactivity disorder with normal controls. *Neurology.* 1997;48:589–601.

Fried PA et al. A follow-up study of attentional behavior in 6-year-old children exposed prenatally to marijuana, cigarettes, and alcohol. *Neurotoxicol Teratol.* 1992;14:299–311.

Grandjean P et al. Cognitive deficit in 7-year-old children with prenatal exposure to methylmercury. *Neurotoxicol Teratol.* 1997;19:417–428.

Greenspan AI, MacKenzie EJ. Functional outcome after pediatric head injury. *Pediatrics.* 1994;94:425–432.

Gross-Tsur V et al. Attention deficit disorder: association with familial-genetic factors. *Pediatr Neurol.* 1991;7:258–261.

Hauser P, Zametkin AJ, Martinez P, et al. Attention deficit-hyperactivity disorder in people with generalized resistance to thyroid hormone. *N Engl J Med.* 1993;328:997–1001.

Holzman C et al. Perinatal brain injury in premature infants born to mothers using alcohol in pregnancy. *Pediatrics.* 1995;95:66–73.

Jacobson JL, Jacobson SW. Intellectual impairment in children exposed to polychlorinated biphenyls in utero. *N Engl J Med.* 1996;335:783–789.

Jones TW et al. Enhanced adrenomedullary response and increased susceptibility to neuroglycopenia: mechanisms underlying the adverse effects of sugar ingestion in healthy children. *J Pediatr.* 1995;126:171–177.

Konofal E, Lecendreux M, Arnulf I, Mouren MC. Iron deficiency in children with attention-deficit/hyperactivity disorder. *Arch Pediatr Adolesc Med*. 2004;158:1113–1115.

Kooistra L et al. Sustained attention problems in children with early treated congenital hypothyroidism. *Acta Paediatr*. 1996;85:425–429.

Krnesi MJP et al. Effects of sugar and aspartame on aggression and activity in children. *Am J Psychiatry*. 1987;144:1487–1490.

Lehn H, Derks EM, Hudziak JJ, Heutink P, van Beijsterveldt TC, Boosma DI. Attention problems and attention-deficit/hypeactivity disorder in discordant and concordant monozygotic twins: evidence of environmental mediators. *J Am Acad Child Adolesc Psychiatry*. 2007; 46:83–91.

Levin HS, Scheller J, Rickard T, et al. Dyscalculia and dyslexia after right hemisphere injury in infancy. *Arch Neurol*. 1996;53:88–96.

Linnet KM, Daisgaard S, Obel C, et al. Maternal lifestyle factors in pregnancy risk of attention-deficit/hyperactivity disorder and associated behaviors: review of the current evidence. *Am J Psychiatry*. 2003;160:1028–1040.

Lopez RE. Hyperactivity in twins. *Can Psychiatr Assoc J*. 1965;10:421.

Lou HC. Etiology and pathogenesis of attention-deficit hyperactivity disorder (ADHD): significance of prematurity and perinatal hypoxic-haemodynamic encephalopathy. *Acta Paediatr*. 1996;85:1266–1271.

Lou HC, Rosa P, Pryds O, et al. ADHD: increased dopamine receptor availability linked to attention deficit and low neonatal cerebral blood flow. *Dev Med Child Neurol*. 2004;46:179–183.

Mahaffey KR. Lead exposure and IQ in children. Editorial. *N Engl J Med*. 1992;327:1308.

Mann CA. Quantitative analysis of EEG in boys with attention-deficit-hyperactivity disorder: controlled study with clinical implications. *Pediatr Neurol*. 1992;8:30–36.

Mataro M et al. Magnetic resonance imaging measurement of the caudate nucleus in adolescents with attention-deficit hyperactivity disorder and its relationship with neuropsychological and behavioral measures. *Arch Neurol*. 1997;54:963–968.

Millichap JG. *The Hyperactive Child with Minimal Brain Dysfunction. Questions and Answers*. Chicago, IL: Year Book; 1975.

Millichap JG. *Nutrition, Diet, and Your Child's Behavior*. Springfield, IL: Charles C Thomas; 1986.

Millichap JG (ed.). *Progress in Pediatric Neurology I, II, & III*. Chicago: PNB Publishers;1991, 1994, & 1997.

Millichap JG. *Environmental Poisons in Our Food*. Chicago: PNB Publishers; 1993.

Millichap JG. *Is Our Water Safe to Drink?* Chicago: PNB Publishers; 1995.

Millichap JG. Temporal lobe arachnoid cyst-attention deficit disorder syndrome. *Neurology*. 1997;48:1435–1439.

Millichap JG. Etiological classification of attention-deficit/hyperactivity disorder. *Pediatrics*. 2008;121:e358–e365.

Millichap JG, Yee MM, Davidson SI. Serum ferritin in children with attention-deficit/hyperactivity disorder. *Pediatr Neurol*. 2006;34:200–203.

Moore BD et al. Neuropsychological significance of areas of high signal intensity on brain MRIs of children with neurofibromatosis. *Neurology*. 1996;46:1660–1668.

Morrison J, Stewart M. The psychiatric status of legal families of adopted hyperactive children. *Arch Gen Psychiatry*. 1973;28:888–891.

Napiorkowski B, Lester BM et al. Effects of in utero substance exposure on infant neurobehavior. *Pediatrics*. 1996;98:71–75.

Niedermeyer E, Naidu SB. Attention-deficit hyperactivity disorder (ADHD) and frontal-motor cortex disconnection. *Clin Electroencephalogr*. 1997;28:130–136.

NIH Consensus Development Conference: Defined diets and childhood hyperactivity. *Clin Pediatr (Phila)*. 1982;21:627–630.

Nordberg L et al. Familial alcoholism and neurobehavior in children. *Acta Paediatr*. 1994;404:14–18,Suppl

Omen GS. Genetic issues in the syndrome of minimal brain dysfunction. In: Walzer S, Wolff PH (eds). *Minimal Cerebral Dysfunction in Children*. New York: Grune & Stratton;1973.

Roizen NJ et al. Psychiatric and developmental disorders in families of children with ADHD. *Arch Pediatr Adolesc Med*. 1996;150:203–208.

Rowe KS. Synthetic food colourings and 'hyperactivity': a double-blind crossover study. *Aust Pediatr*. 1988;24:143–147.

Safer DJ. The familial incidence of minimal brain dysfunction. In: Wender PH. *Minimal Brain Dysfunction in Children*. New York: Wiley-Interscience; 1969, 1971.Unpublished study.

Scafidi FA, Field TM et al. Cocaine-exposed preterm neonates show behavioral and hormonal differences. *Pediatrics*. 1996;97:851–855.

Schantz SI. Developmental neurotoxicity of polychlorinated biphenyls (PCBs) in humans. *Neurotoxicol Teratol*. 1996;18:217–227.

Segal MM, Rogers GF, Needleman HL, Chapman CA. Hypokalemic sensory overstimulation. *J Child Neurol*. 2007;22:1408–1410.

Shaywitz BA et al. Aspartame, behavior, and cognitive function in children with attention deficit disorder. *Pediatrics*. 1994;93:70–75.

Sherman DK et al. Attention-deficit hyperactivity disorder dimensions: a twin study of inattention and impulsivity-hyperactivity. *J Am Acad Child Adolesc Psychiatry*. 1997;36:745–753.

Smalley SL. Behavioral genetics '97. Genetic influences in childhood-onset psychiatric disorders: autism and attention deficit/hyperactivity disorder. *Am J Hum Genet*. 1997;60:1276–1282.

St Sauver JL, Barbaresi WJ, Katusic SK, Colligan RC, Weaver AL, Jacobsen SJ. Early life risk factors for attention-deficit/hyperactivity disorder: a population-based cohort study. *Mayo Clin Proc*. 2004;79:1124–1131.

Suresh PA, Sebastian S, George A, Radhakrishnan K. Subclinical hyperthyroidism and hyperkinetic behavior in children. *Pediatr Neurol*. 1999;20:192–194.

Swanson JM, Kinsbourne M, Nigg J, et al. Etiologic subtypes of attention-deficit/hyperactivity disorder: brain imaging, molecular genetic and environmental factors and the dopamine hypothesis. *Neuropsychol Rev*. 2007;17:39–59.

Thapar A, Langley K, Asherson P, Gill M. Gene-environment interplay in attention-deficit hyperactivity disorder and the importance of a developmental perspective. *Br J Psychiatry*. 2007;190:1–3.

Tiwari BD, Godbole MM et al. Learning disabilities and poor motivation to achieve due to prolonged iodine deficiency. *Am J Clin Nutr*. 1996;63:782–786.

Tronick EZ et al. Late dose-response effects of prenatal cocaine exposure on neurobehavioral performance. *Pediatrics*. 1996;98:76–83.

Valdimarsdottir M, Hrafnsdottir AH, Magnusson P, Gudmundsson OO. The frequency of some factors in pregnancy and delivery for Icelandic children with ADHD [in Icelandic]. *Laeknabladid*. 2006;92:609–614.

Vermiglio F, Lo Presti VP, Moleti M, et al. Attention deficit and hyperactivity disorders in the offspring of mothers exposed to mild-moderate iodine deficiency: a possible novel iodine deficiency disorder in developed countries. *J Clin Endocrinol Metab*. 2004;89:6054–6060.

Voeller KKS. The neurological basis of attention deficit hyperactivity disorder. *Int Pediatr*. 1990;5:171–176.

Weiss RE, Stein MA, Trommer B, Refetoff S. Attention-deficit hyperactivity disorder and thyroid function. *J Pediatr*. 1993;123:539–545.

Wender EH, Solanto MV. Effects of sugar on aggressive and inattentive behavior in children with attention deficit disorder with hyperactivity and normal children. *Pediatrics*. 1991;88:960–966.

Whitaker AH et al. Psychiatric outcomes in low-birth-weight children at age 6 years: relation to neonatal cranial ultrasound abnormalities. *Arch Gen Psychiatry*. 1997;54:847–856.

Wolraich ML, Wilson DB, White JW. The effect of sugar on behavior or cognition in children. A *meta-analysis*. *JAMA*. 1995;274:1617–1621.

Wrightson P et al. Mild head injury in preschool children: Evidence that it can be associated with a persisting cognitive defect. *J Neurol Neurosurg Psychiatry*. 1995;59:375–380.

Yehuda S. Brain biochemistry and behavior. *Nutr Rev*. 1986;44:1–250,Supplement May

Yehuda S. Effects of dietary nutrients and deficiencies on brain biochemistry and behavior. *Int J Neurosci*. 1987;35:21–36.

Zametkin AJ, Rapoport JL. Neurobiology of attention deficit disorder with hyperactivity: where have we come in 50 years? *J Am Acad Child Adolesc Psychiatry*. 1987;26:676–686.

Chapter 3
Symptoms and Signs of ADHD

The symptoms of ADHD are outlined in the DSM-IV diagnostic criteria in two main subtypes or groups: (1) symptoms of inattentiveness and (2) hyperactivity-impulsivity. Signs of brain dysfunction and associated perceptual and learning disabilities are omitted from the current definition, as outlined by the American Psychiatric Association. The recognition of both symptoms and signs of ADHD is important, however, particularly in terms of defining the cause and treatment.

ADHD as defined by the DSM-IV rarely occurs alone. Certain neuropsychiatric disorders frequently complicate the diagnosis of ADHD and often modify the treatment. Many of these disorders are neurological, including headache, seizures, tics or Tourette syndrome, and speech and language and motor coordination problems. Others are psychiatric or neuropsychological in nature, principally oppositional defiance disorder (ODD), conduct disorder (CD), and learning disorders.

The differential diagnosis, or conditions that may present with some of the symptoms of ADHD, includes bipolar disorders (depression, dysthymia), pervasive developmental disorders (autism, Asperger's syndrome), personality disorders (obsessive compulsive disorder (OCD)), and mental retardation syndromes. The physician who treats children with ADHD needs to be familiar with associated disorders that may require investigation and specialized methods of management.

Occasional "Inattentiveness" or an "Attention Deficit Disorder"?

Most children have periods of "day dreaming" in school when attention wanders transiently, but not sufficiently to impair learning. Inattentiveness becomes an attention deficit disorder (ADD) when the child is unable to sustain attention and is frequently distracted by outside stimuli. In order to attend, the child must ignore or tune out irrelevant distracting stimuli. The child with ADD fails to inhibit the background "noise" in the classroom environment (Rosenberger, 1991). Symptoms of ADD also include a listening problem, forgetfulness, weakness in organization, and inability to complete a task.

J.G. Millichap, *Attention Deficit Hyperactivity Disorder Handbook*, DOI 10.1007/978-1-4419-1397-5_3, © Springer Science+Business Media, LLC 2010

If the inattentiveness is episodic and the child appears confused, the possibility of absence or partial complex seizures is considered and an electroencephalogram (EEG) is recommended. The distinction between a sustained inattentiveness, characteristic of ADD, and seizures is important in determining the medical management. Stimulant medication prescribed for ADD may worsen the episodes of inattention related to a seizure disorder. A non-stimulant medication is often preferred for children with ADD and an abnormal EEG.

Measurement of Attention

Measures of attention involve the direct observation of the child or the indirect questioning of parents and teachers. Direct measures of attention are of three types: (1) recording the alpha rhythm on the EEG and by evoked potentials (EP); (2) tests of reaction time, continuous performance tests, paired associated learning, and tests of memorization; and (3) psychometric tests such as the WISC, Stanford-Binet, Detroit, and Reading achievement. Measures 1 and 2 are mainly relevant in research and have little application in clinical practice. The EEG alpha activity (8–13 Hz) reflects a state of relaxation and inattention to the environment; beta activity (14–25 Hz) is activated by emotional and cognitive processes (Ray and Cole, 1985).

Computerized quantitative analysis of the EEG, performed in 25 boys with ADHD compared to 27 matched controls, showed a decrease in beta and an increase in theta (4–7 Hz) activity. Differences were enhanced in ADHD subjects during reading and drawing tasks, especially in frontal areas of the head (Mann, 1992). Increases in the latency of the P300 wave, an evoked response generated by attention, correlates with cognitive impairment (Finley et al., 1985).

Reaction time has been used to demonstrate attentiveness and cognitive improvement after stimulant therapy (Sprague et al., 1970). Divided attention to multiple stimuli has been monitored by reinforcement, using operant conditioning to study visual inattention in subjects with parietal lobe damage (Rosenberger, 1974). The continuous performance test (CPT), using errors of commission or omission as measures of inattention to change of stimuli and impulsivity, is complex and allows some children to compensate for an AD (Trommer et al., 1988). The paired associate learning (PAL) test, using the coding or digit symbol subtest of the WISC, is sensitive to the inattention and distractibility of the learning-disabled child with ADHD (Kinsbourne and Conners, 1990), as are standard memory tests.

Learning requires attention, and psychometric measures of cognitive function are sensitive to inattention. Analysis of the WISC intelligence subtests – arithmetic, digit span, and coding – demonstrates relatively low scores in hyperactive children, a reflection of the adverse effects of inattention and distractibility on learning. Attention deficit interferes with the performance of several additional tests of intelligence and short-term memory: the Stroop Color and Word Test, the Stanford-Binet Intelligence Scale, the Detroit Test of Learning Aptitudes, and the MacGinitie Reading Test. Neuropsychological testing is an essential part of the investigation of the child with ADHD.

The Conners questionnaire (1969) is the earliest and most widely used measure of attention deficit in children with ADHD. Parent and teacher questionnaires are either short or long. They usually use a 4-point rating system, and they distinguish the factors of hyperactivity, inattention, impulsivity, and peer interaction.

When Is Hyperactivity Abnormal?

Children normally have an excessive degree of motor restlessness at times, particularly in emotionally charged environments. Hyperactive behavior is abnormal when accompanied by short attention span and distractibility, and when it is purposeless, inappropriate and undirected toward a specific, meaningful goal. The inability to focus and perform structured tasks is the hallmark of the hyperactive school-age child. The quality and direction of the hyperactivity are abnormal, not necessarily the total daily activity. Hyperactivity is frequently accompanied by impulsivity, a tendency to interrupt others and inability to wait in line.

The child with ADHD is often restless in infancy. As a toddler, "he is into everything," and has to be watched constantly for his own protection and that of household breakables. In later childhood, he is constantly fidgeting, always "on the go," and is unable to sit still at the dinner table. At school, the teacher also reports an inability to sit still; he gets up and walks around in the classroom, he talks excessively, interrupts, and tends to distract and disturb others. The motor hyperactivity is often accompanied by "verbal hyperactivity," and sometimes a flight of ideas, without focus on the topic of conversation.

In anatomical studies of the origin of hyperactivity, two types are distinguished: (1) *overreactivity* caused by frontal lobe injury and a response to external environmental stimulation; and (2) *essential overactivity* caused by striatal lesions and a release of motor activity normally inhibited by frontal-striatal connections in the brain (Magoun, 1963; Millichap, 1997). We may infer that some children with ADHD are overreactive only when stimulated by a noisy environment, whereas others exhibit a constant uninhibited motor activity unrelated to the environment. The hyperactivity may appear normal in the playground but abnormal and inappropriate in the classroom.

Devices Used to Measure Motor Activity

Several methods have been used experimentally to measure the degree of motor activity. These include the pedometer, to quantify gross locomotor activity; a stabilimetric cushion, to record the degree of wiggling or fidgeting; and a grid-marked floor, which permits assessment of the time spent in one activity or the degree of mobility from one location in a room to another. The author has used a device called an "actometer," an automatically winding calendar wrist-watch with the pendulum connected directly to the hands, so that movements of either arms or legs may be recorded in minutes and hours. The actometer was used in some early controlled studies of the effects of methylphenidate in the treatment of ADHD (Millichap et al., 1968). A device similar to the "actometer," and called an "actigraph," a wristwatch-sized recorder worn on a belt, is now available.

More recently, an infrared video and motion analysis system was used to record movement patterns of boys with ADHD and normal controls during a continuous performance task (CPT) (Teicher et al., 1996). Compared to controls, subjects with ADHD moved their extremities and head more than twice as often, and they covered a threefold greater distance and a fourfold greater area. Whole body movements were also 3–4 times more frequent. Responses on the CPT were slower and more variable. The movement patterns of ADHD children correlated with the teacher ratings of hyperactivity and inattention.

These objective measures of motor activity are of value in experimental situations, particularly in trials of new medical treatments. They may also be indicated for the confirmation of diagnosis of overactivity when parent and teacher impressions are in disagreement. From a practical standpoint in the everyday management of the child with ADHD they are of limited value.

"Subtle" or "Soft" Neurological Signs

Mild or subtle neurologic abnormalities are sometimes referred to as "soft" signs. Many children with ADHD are described as clumsy or uncoordinated. They may be poor at sports, especially basketball and activities requiring a quick reaction and facile movements. Soft signs are usually indicative of immaturity or delayed development of the nervous system. Sometimes, the clumsiness and signs will persist into adult life. Unlike cerebral palsy, the incoordination of movement is not associated with obvious muscle weakness or spasticity. Movements (synkinetic or mirror) that are normally inhibited by 5–7 years of age persist into older age groups, and coordination abilities (hopping and tandem gait) usually accomplished by five years are delayed. In eliciting motor function, the speed, overflow, and rhythm of movement are important characteristics of subtle neurological abnormalities. Timed repetitive finger tapping, foot-to-hand overflow in tandem gait, and failure to maintain a steady rhythm of motor movement are examples used in quantitative tests of neurological assessment of subtle signs (Denckla, 1985).

Motor impersistence is a characteristic neurological soft sign of ADHD. The term was first coined to describe the difficulty in maintaining a motor behavior experienced by brain injured adults, even though they had no problem in initiating or performing the movements. The injury was located in the right hemisphere of the brain, especially the frontal lobe, an area often involved in ADHD. Motor impersistence is manifested by an inability to maintain movements such as the following on request: "close your eyes," "look at my nose or finger," "put out your tongue," or "hold your arms outstretched."

Response inhibition deficit. In addition to motor impersistence, the child with ADHD demonstrates an inability to inhibit responses. A child will be unable to look away from a stimulus when requested. When asked to hold out the arms and stand still, he will frequently initiate other movements such as walking. The teacher will complain, "he can't keep his hands to himself." If he sees a pencil or a pair of scissors, he is unable to look at the object without putting it to its intended use, a sign of "utilization behavior." Deficits in response inhibition are a reflection of inattentiveness, the tendency to respond to distracting stimuli, and of impulsivity (Voeller, 1990).

Dyspraxia or *apraxia* is another soft neurologic sign commonly recognized in association with ADHD. Dyspraxia is a loss or delayed development of dexterity in purposeful movements, as in hopping, tandem walking, or the use of scissors, despite normal muscle strength. The term dyspraxia is also applied to an inability to protrude the tongue on command, yet the movement is carried out involuntarily. A delay in speech may be a form of apraxia. A constructional apraxia is an inability to build blocks or copy simple designs. Dyspraxias are caused by dysfunction or damage to the frontal lobes of the brain.

Dysdiadochokinesia is the neurological term for clumsiness in the performance of rapidly alternating movements (pronation and supination) of the forearms. Children aged 5–7 years should be able to imitate the examiner's movements without mirroring the movement in the opposite forearm. Involuntary mirror movements are referred to as *synkinesia,* and are a common sign of minimal brain dysfunction in ADHD. When the child is older he is usually able to inhibit these mirror movements.

Ataxia and incoordination, also described as clumsiness, may represent an immaturity or damage to the cerebellum and its connections. An attempt to walk a straight line is performed unsteadily, and finger-to-nose movements of the upper limbs bring out a tremor.

Choreiform movements are involuntary jerky movements, usually demonstrated by asking the child to stretch out his arms. Prechtl and Stemmer (1962) reported choreiform movements as a sign of minimal brain dysfunction, an earlier term for ADHD. In my experience, choreiform movements are uncommon and not a characteristic sign associated with ADHD. They should not be regarded as "soft" signs.

Graphanesthesia, an inability to recognize numerals traced on the skin of the palms or the back, is a common finding with ADHD. It is indicative of dysfunction of the parietal lobes of the brain.

Other neurological signs sometimes elicited include a tendency to walk on the toes due to tight heel cords or contractures of the Achilles tendons, and Babinski signs, an extension of the great toe and fanning of the second to the fifth toes when the plantar surface of the foot is stroked with a blunt object. These signs are not included under the term "soft" neurological abnormalities, since they commonly persist and may be evidence of permanent dysfunction of the pyramidal tracts and cerebrospinal motor system.

Soft neurological signs were of predictive value for learning disabilities in preschool children, aged 3–5 years, in a study at the *Wyler Children's Hospital,*

University of Chicago, IL (Huttenlocher et al., 1990). A poor neurological test score at age five correlated with a lower Full-scale IQ at age seven. Neurologic soft signs accurately identified nearly all the children who needed special educational help. Abnormal neurologic signs identical to those included in the above test battery were previously correlated with hyperactive behavior, ADHD, and a beneficial response to stimulant medication, in a study at *Northwestern University Medical School, Chicago* (Millichap, 1974).

Gender differences in age-related changes in subtle motor signs are documented in 132 children with ADHD and 136 normal controls, in a study at *Johns Hopkins University School of Medicine, Baltimore, MD* (Cole et al., 2008). Both controls and ADHD groups showed improvement on timed tasks (e.g. finger-tapping) with age, although ADHD children were relatively slower across the age span of 7–14 years. Whereas controls and girls with ADHD showed steady age-related reduction of foot-to-hand overflow and dysrhythmia (failure to maintain steady rhythm), boys with ADHD showed little improvement in these signs through age 14 years. These changes in "soft" neurological signs pattern findings in brain neuroimaging studies, in which anomalies in motor control areas are more prominent in boys than girls with ADHD. The gender differences may be related to earlier brain maturation in girls.

A careful examination and recording of neurological abnormalities help in our understanding of the causes and anatomical lesions in the brain that may explain the mechanism of ADHD. The need for special diagnostic laboratory investigations such as EEG and MRI is determined by the neurological history and examination findings.

Developmental Coordination Disorder Diagnostic Criteria

Incoordination is a frequent abnormality elicited on neurological examination of the child with ADHD. In the Diagnostic and Statistical Manual of Mental Disorders: DSM-IV criteria (1994), coordination disorders are labeled as *Developmental Coordination Disorder* (200.80) or DCD. The diagnostic criteria for DCD are summarized as follows:

A. Delays in achieving motor milestones, clumsiness, poor sports performance, or poor handwriting.
B. Incoordination significantly interferes with academic achievement or activities of daily living.
C. The disorder is not due to cerebral palsy, muscular dystrophy, or other medical illness and does not meet criteria for a Pervasive Developmental Disorder.

The association of coordination problems with ADHD and especially with hyperactive behavior is described under the terms *minimal brain dysfunction* (Clements, 1966) and *DAMP syndrome* (Landgren et al., 2000). Minimal brain dysfunction

(MBD) was a term used to describe children of near or above average intelligence, with learning and/or behavioral abnormalities associated with subtle deviations of CNS function. The definition of MBD included deficits in coordination, perception, conceptualization, language, memory and control of attention, and impulse or motor function (Millichap, 1977). DAMP, a Scandinavian syndrome, includes deficits in attention, motor control, and perception. The terms MBD and DAMP are inclusive of patients with ADHD, DCD and learning disabilities, whereas ADHD is a symptom only diagnosis that fails to recognize frequently associated coordination and perceptual dysfunction.

Relation Between Motor Performance and ADHD

In a study of 42 school-aged children with ADHD at the *National Taiwan University*, the performance in fine and gross motor skills was significantly impaired, as measured by the Bruininks-Oseretsky Test of Motor Proficiency and compared to 42 age- and sex-matched children without ADHD. (Tseng et al., 2004). Sustained attention and impulse control are important predictors of both fine and gross motor skills. Hyperactivity is a predictor of gross motor incoordination but is not significantly correlated with fine motor skills. Based on the frequency of subtle neurological abnormalities in children with ADHD and impaired motor performance, a primary motor deficit is a more likely explanation than motor incoordination secondary to impaired attention and lack of impulse (inhibitory) control.

These studies indicate that measures of motor performance should be included in the diagnostic criteria for ADHD. In the next edition of DSM criteria, perhaps a subtype of ADH and Incoordination Disorder (ADHID) would be appropriate.

Summary

Symptoms of ADHD as outlined in the DSM-IV criteria are in 2 groups or subtypes, inattentiveness and hyperactivity-impulsiveness. Signs of brain dysfunction frequently associated, such as coordination, perceptual and learning disabilities, are omitted from the current definition of the syndrome.

Inattentiveness becomes an attention deficit disorder when the child is unable to sustain attention and is frequently distracted. Hyperactive behavior is abnormal when accompanied by short attention span and distractibility, and when purposeless, inappropriate and undirected toward a specific, meaningful goal. Inability to focus and perform structured tasks is the hallmark of the school-age child with ADHD.

Many children with ADHD are described as clumsy and having signs of developmental coordination disorder. Neurological examination will often uncover subtle abnormalities, referred to as "soft" signs. These may be indicative of a delayed maturity of the central nervous system, and improvement is expected with increasing age, especially in girls. Soft neurological signs are predictive of learning disabilities and are correlated with hyperactive behavior, inattention, and a beneficial response to stimulant medication.

References

American Psychiatric Association. *Diagnostic and Statistical Manual of Mental Disorders*. 4th ed. Wasshington, DC: American Psychiatric Association; 1994.

Clements SD. Minimal brain dysfunction in children. NINDS Monograph No. 3, US Public Health Service Bulletin No. 1415, Washington, DC, US Department of Health, Education, and Welfare; 1966.

Cole WR, Mostofsky SH, Larson JCG, Denckla MB, Mahone EM. Age-related changes in motor subtle signs among girls and boys with ADHD. *Neurology*. 2008;71:1514–1520.

Conners C. A teacher rating scale for use in drug studies with children. *Am J Psychiatry*. 1969;126:152–156.

Denckla MB. Revised neurological examination for subtle signs. *Psychopharmacol Bull*. 1985;21:773–779.

Finley W, et al. Long-latency event-related potentials in the evaluation of cognitive function in children. *Neurology*. 1985;35:323–327.

Huttenlocher PR, Levine SC, Huttenlocher J, Gates J. Discrimination of normal and at-risk preschool children on the basis of neurological tests. *Dev Med Child Neurol*. 1990;32:394–402.

Kinsbourne M, Conners C eds. *Diagnosis and Treatment of Attention Deficit Disorders*. Munich: MMW Press; 1990.

Landgren M, Kjellman B, Gillberg C. Deficits in attention, motor control and perception (DAMP): a simplified school entry examination. *Acta Paediatr*. 2000;89:302–309.

Magoun HW. *The Waking Brain*. 2nd ed. Springfield, IL: Charles C Thomas; 1963.

Mann CA. Quantitative analysis of EEG in boys with attention-deficit-hyperactivity disorder: controlled study with clinical implications. *Pediatr Neurol*. 1992;8:30–36.

Millichap JG, et al. Hyperactive behavior and learning disorders: battery of neuropsychological tests in controlled trial of methylphenidate. *Am J Dis Child*. 1968;116:237–244.

Millichap JG. Methylphenidate in hyperkinetic behavior: relation of response to degree of activity and brain damage. In: Conners CK, ed. *Clinical Use of Stimulant Drugs in Children*. Amsterdam: Excerpta Medica; 1974.

Millichap JG. Definitions and diagnosis of minimal brain dysfunction. In Millichap JG, ed. *Learning Disabilities and Related Disorders: Facts and Current Issues*. Chicago, IL: Year Book Medical Publishers; 1977:3–11.

Millichap JG. Organic theory of ADHD. In Millichap JG, ed. *Progress in Pediatric Neurology Vol III*. Chicago, IL: PNB Publishers; 1997:198–201.

Prechtl HFR, Stemmer C. The choreiform syndrome in children. *Dev Med Child Neurol*. 1962;4:119.

Ray W, Cole H. EEG alpha activity reflects attentional demands and beta activity reflects emotional and cognitive processes. *Science*. 1985;228:750–752.

Rosenberger PB. Discriminative aspects of visual hemi-inattention. *Neurology*. 1974;24:18–23.

Rosenberger PB. Attention deficit. *Pediatr Neurol*. 1991;7:397–405.

Sprague R, et al. Methylphenidate and thioridiazine: learning, reaction time, activity, and classroom behavior in disturbed children. *Am J Orthopsychiatry*. 1970;40:615–628.

Teicher MH, et al. Objective measurement of hyperactivity and attentional problems in ADHD. *J Am Acad Child Adolesc Psychiatry*. 1996;35:334–342.

Trommer BL, et al. Pitfalls in the use of a continuous performance test as a diagnostic tool in attention deficit disorder. *J Dev Behav Pediatr*. 1988;9:339–346.

Tseng MH, Henderson A, Chow SMK, Yao G. Relationship between motor proficiency, attention, impulse, and activity in children with ADHD. *Dev Med Child Neurol*. 2004;46:381–388.

Voeller KKS. The neurological basis of attention deficit hyperactivity disorder. *Int Pediatr*. 1990;5:171–176.

Chapter 4
Diagnosis and Laboratory Tests

The diagnosis of ADHD is determined by an evaluation of reports from parents and teachers and by observation and examination of the child in the office of the physician or psychologist. The parents and teachers should provide completed questionnaires that rate attention, behavior, impulsivity, academic achievement, and social skills. Since the symptoms of ADHD are especially troublesome when the child enters school, the teacher is often the first to draw attention to the problem and advise the parents to consult their pediatrician.

Significance of History and Examination

The history of pregnancy, birth, and early development may uncover abnormalities indicative of prenatal, perinatal, or postnatal disorders with etiological significance in ADHD. Examples are viral infection and exposure to nicotine during pregnancy, anoxia and prematurity at birth, and trauma, toxins and infection in neonatal and infantile periods. The family history may suggest genetic factors in etiology or susceptibility to comorbid disorders (e.g. conduct disorder, tics, seizures, migraine headache, or learning disorders) or a tendency to heart irregularities, important in the management of stimulant medications. The reports of achievements and difficulties in preschool, kindergarten, and grade school will be evaluated. The history taking is followed by general physical and neurological examinations. Schoolteacher reports and any tests previously ordered by the pediatrician, family practitioner, or psychologist are reviewed. The response to previous treatments is recorded.

Genetic and environmental causes will be considered and the need for special tests determined. The indications for EEG, MRI, blood analyses, chromosome studies, and neuropsychological evaluation are reviewed. After all criteria for the diagnosis of ADHD and complicating medical conditions have been determined and considered, the pros and cons of stimulant or other types of medication are discussed..

J.G. Millichap, *Attention Deficit Hyperactivity Disorder Handbook*,
DOI 10.1007/978-1-4419-1397-5_4, © Springer Science+Business Media, LLC 2010

Questions Asked of Parent in Making ADHD Diagnosis

A parent should be prepared to answer the following questions at a pediatric or pediatric neurology consultation:

- What are your main concerns and when did the symptoms begin? Are the hyperactivity and/or inattentiveness present both in the home and at school?
- What is your child's grade placement, the number of pupils in the class, the type of school, and is the education bilingual? Were any grades repeated?
- Has the teacher suggested the consultation and did you bring a written report or completed questionnaire regarding behavior, attention, and achievement?
- Was the mother well during the pregnancy or did she suffer from infection, diabetes, or trauma, or use alcohol, tobacco, or drugs? Does she take thyroid hormone?
- Was the birth normal or complicated? What was the birth weight? Was the birth premature? What were the Apgar scores or vital signs at birth? Did the baby breathe normally or need resuscitation? Did jaundice develop and require treatment? How long was the baby in the hospital?
- What were the milestones of early development? Did the child walk by 14 months, talk in short phrases by 2 years, pedal a tricycle by 3 years, and know colors by 5 years?
- Is there any history of seizures, fever convulsions, episodic daydreaming or confused appearance, headaches, sleep disorders, enuresis, head trauma, tics, ear infections, cardiac problem, asthma, or illness requiring chronic medication?
- Have vision and hearing been checked? Has the blood lead level been tested?
- Does your child exhibit any other behavioral problems that sometimes complicate ADHD, such as oppositional defiance or conduct disorder?
- Do other members of the family have a history of ADHD or related neuropsychiatric problems? Are there siblings, and what are their ages and academic placements and achievements? What is the health and occupation of the parents? Does any family member have a history of cardiac or thyroid disease? Is the family environment supportive or divided?
- How do the parents view the need and acceptance of medication, if treatment is recommended?

Physical and Neurological Examinations

The general physical examination includes measurements of head circumference, height and weight, vision and hearing, heart sounds and blood pressure, birthmarks and congenital developmental anomalies or dysmorphisms. The neurological examination should test for subtle neurological abnormalities or soft signs, including dyspraxias of gait and incoordination, dysdiadochokinesia, mirror movements, motor impersistence, graphanesthesia, handwriting problems, handedness, right–left disorientation, finger agnosia, dyscalculia, reading disorder, and speech and language delay. The recognition of subtle neurological abnormalities is an indication of delayed maturation or complicating visual perception and learning disorders. These findings may impact the response to treatment and outcome of ADHD.

For further details of the pediatric neurological examination see the following: Gordon (1993), Menkes (1985), Millichap (1991), Paine and Oppe (1966), and Swaiman (1994).

Indications for an EEG in Children with ADHD

An EEG may be considered in the following circumstances:

- History of frequent "daydreaming" or episodic lack of awareness;
- Personal or family history of epilepsy, as a precursor to treatment with stimulants that may precipitate seizures in susceptible patients;
- ADHD complicated by language delay.

Indications for an MRI or CT Scan in a Child with ADHD

MRI or CT scan of the head is indicated for the following complications:

- Headaches with symptoms of increased intracranial pressure or signs of structural brain lesion;
- Seizures and an abnormal EEG showing focal epileptiform discharge or focal slowing;
- ADHD complicated by language delay and seizures;
- ADHD and learning disability associated with neurocutaneous syndromes (e.g. neurofibromatosis, Sturge-Weber syndrome).

Blood Tests Sometimes Indicated in ADHD

Routine laboratory tests are not recommended in the American Academy of Pediatrics Clinical Practice Guideline (AAP, 2000). Blood tests sometimes helpful in determining the cause or contributing factors in ADHD include the following:

- CBC to rule out anemia and iron deficiency;
- Serum ferritin, a measure of iron storage;
- Blood lead level, especially in younger children with higher risks of exposure;
- Liver function tests as preliminary to treating ADHD with drugs that sometimes elevate liver enzymes;
- Thyroid profile, free T4 and TSH, to rule out thyroid dysfunction, especially in children of short stature or having a family history of thyroid disease;
- Chromosome analysis, especially in children with signs of fragile X disease or signs of developmental defect.

Indications for Electrocardiogram and/or Cardiac Consult

Need for cardiovascular risk screening before starting stimulant medication in children with ADHD is controversial. The American Heart Association advises routine pretreatment electrocardiogram (ECG) whereas the American Academy of Pediatrics considers routine ECG to be unnecessary. Cardiac history and examination are recommended, and ECG and cardiac consultation, only if clinically indicated (Perrin et al., 2008).

A *full cardiac screen* consists of all of the following:

● History of congenital or other heart disease?
● Family history of sudden death?
● Family history of early coronary infarct?
● Record of pulse and blood pressure;
● Examination for heart murmur;
● Obtain ECG.

Modified cardiac screen is the same as above, except the ECG is performed selectively for children with heart murmur or other cardiac abnormality.

Pretreatment ECG conservative indications are suggested as follows:

● Heart murmur;
● Abnormal blood pressure and/or pulse irregularity;
● Personal or family history of early heart disease;
● Involvement in competitive sports.

ECG indications during treatment with medications for ADHD:

● Complaint of chest pain or shortness of breath during exercise;
● Abnormalities of pulse or blood pressure;
● Heart murmur;
● Use of higher doses of medication.

Cardiac consultation and echocardiogram are recommended if the ECG is abnormal or heart murmur is detected. The decision to refer for cardiac consultation is dependent on the treating physician's expertise. The cardiologist may clear the patient for stimulant medications, but the treating physician makes the final decision to treat or not to treat.

Canadian practice policies. Since *Health Canada* released a statement advising against stimulants in ADHD patients with cardiac disease in May 2006, after isolated reports of sudden death, physicians' assessment and treatment of ADHD patients have changed (Conway et al., 2008). The proportion performing a full cardiac screen increased for both noncardiologists (0.2–15.1%) and cardiologists (54.8–68.6%) after the advisory. The change in the use of a modified screen was 7.4–34.5% for noncardiologists and no increase for cardiologists (7.8–5.9%). The proportion of noncardiologists willing to prescribe stimulant medications in children with potential or actual cardiac issues showed a considerable decrease. The changes in practice following the advisory occurred despite the lack of studies to address the actual cardiac risks of stimulant medication. Consensus recommendations are required to determine the necessity for pretreatment screening and to establish significant risk factors for cardiac complications of ADHD treatment.

Tests of Research Interest Only

Parents sometimes ask about tests used principally in research studies at university centers. These include positron emission tomography (PET) and SPECT, tests used to demonstrate changes in glucose metabolism in the frontal lobes of patients with ADHD. The tests involve isotopes and are not generally advised in children.

Brainstem auditory evoked potentials (BAEPs) or responses (BAERs) show changes that may be used as tests for ADD and the differentiation of ADHD subtypes. Evoked potentials and quantitative EEG analysis have also been used to study cognitive impairments. Research-orientated laboratories are required for these types of studies and the evaluation of results.

Quantitative MRI may demonstrate volumetric changes in the brain, and *functional MRI (fMRI)* measures brain cell activity in various cerebral locations, tests of value in investigating the cause and brain localization of ADHD and learning disabilities.

Magnetoencephalography (MEG) may be used to track brain activation sequences during reading. MEG records the magnetic effects of the EEG currents during brain activation, a spatial-temporal measuring device.

Blood, urine, and spinal fluid measurements of neurotransmitters, norepinephrine, and dopamine show changes in some patients with ADHD, and these are modified by treatment with methylphenidate. The biochemical basis for ADHD is an interesting research topic but insufficiently documented for use in practice.

Early Risk Factors for a Diagnosis of ADHD in Childhood

The following factors may be predictive of the early development of ADHD before a child enters kindergarten:

- Family history of ADHD;
- Maternal smoking or drinking alcohol during pregnancy;
- A mother addicted to cocaine during the pregnancy and neonatal period;
- Poor socio-economic status and low educational attainment of parents;
- Exposure to lead and elevated blood lead levels in infancy and early childhood;
- Delayed milestones of speech and language and psychomotor development (see Table 4.1);

Table 4.1 Milestones of development in infancy and early childhood

Age	Motor function	Communication
1 month	Infantile grasp reflex; reflex stepping	Blinks to light; startles with noise
4 months	Good head control; shakes rattle	Follows fully with eyes; turns to sound, smiles
6 months	Transfers objects; rolls over on back	Extends arms to be held; responds to name
8 months	Sits without support	Says "da-da" sounds
9 months	Crawls; stands with support; picks up crumb with thumb and finger	Plays "patty-cake"; waves "bye-bye"; responds to "no"
12 months	Walks, one hand held	Knows 2–4 words
14 months	Walks alone	Builds 2 block tower
18 months	Feeds self	Many single words
2 years	Runs, kicks ball; bunny hops	2–3-word sentences; knows name
3 years	Rides tricycle	Copies circle
4 years	Walks up stairs	Copies cross
5 years	Walks tandem; hops on one foot	Copies square; knows colors
6 years	Rides bicycle	Copies triangle
7 years		Copies diamond

- Evidence of hyperactivity and irritability during infancy;
- Exposure to unstructured and critical discipline practices and unstable emotional climate in the home.

Summary

The diagnosis of ADHD is dependent on reports of parents and teachers regarding a child's behavior, attention and academic progress, and a physician or psychologist's examination. The examination should include the history of birth and early development, family history, physical and neurological signs, and reports of psychological tests. Routine laboratory tests are not recommended. Special tests with specific indications include an electroencephalogram, electrocardiogram, magnetic resonance imaging of the brain, blood lead, serum ferritin, thyroid profile, CBC, liver function, and chromosome analysis. The American Academy of Pediatrics Guideline provides a useful framework for the diagnostic evaluation, but clinical judgment should determine the appropriate approach for the individual child with ADHD.

References

American Academy of Pediatrics. Clinical practice guideline: diagnosis and evaluation of the child with attention-deficit/hyperactivity disorder. *Pediatrics*. 2000;105:1158–1170.

Conway J, Wong KK, O'Connell C, Warren AE. Cardiovascular risk screening before starting stimulant medications and prescribing practices of Canadian physicians: Impact of the Health Canada Advisory. *Pediatrics*. 2008;122:e828–e834.

Gordon N. *Neurological Problems in Childhood*. Oxford: Butterworth-Heinemann; 1993.

Menkes JH. *Textbook of Child Neurology*. 3rd ed.. Philadelphia, PA: Lea & Febiger; 1985.

Millichap JG Ed.. *Progress in Pediatric Neurology I, II, & III*. Chicago, IL: PNB Publishers; 1991:94 & 97.

Paine RS, Oppe TE. *Neurologic Examination of Children*. Clin Dev Med Vol. 20/21. Oxford: Spastics Society and Heinemann Med Publ; 1966.

Perrin JM, et al. . *Pediatrics*. 2008;12:451–453.

Swaiman KF. *Pediatric Neurology. Principles and Practice*. 2nd ed, Vol 1. St Louis, MO: Mosby; 1994.

Chapter 5
Oppositional, Conduct, and Other ADHD Comorbid Disorders

Psychiatric disorders sometimes associated with ADHD include oppositional defiant disorder, conduct disorder, mood disorders, and anxiety disorders, including obsessive compulsive disorder. These are referred to as comorbid disorders. They complicate the management of ADHD and, if severe enough to impair school and social functioning, will require psychiatric or psychological intervention. For practical purposes, the following definitions are simplified from the DSM-IV diagnostic criteria.

Oppositional Defiant Disorder

The criteria for the diagnosis of oppositional defiant disorder include at least five of the following, present for at least six months:

- Loses temper often
- Argues with adults
- Refuses to do chores
- Annoys other people
- Blames others
- Easily annoyed
- Often angry
- Often spiteful
- Swears frequently

Conduct Disorder

A conduct disorder is significant if at least three of the following criteria have been present for at least six months:

- Steals
- Runs away from home

- Lies
- Sets fires
- Plays truant
- Breaks into someone's house, building, or car
- Destroys others property
- Cruel to animals and/or people
- Sexually abusive
- Starts fights, with or without a weapon

Mood Disorders

Mood disorders sometimes complicating ADHD include manic and/or depressive episodes, bipolar disorders, cyclothymia, and dysthymia.

A *manic episode* consists of elevated or irritable mood sufficient to impair school and social functioning and associated with at least three of the following:

- Heightened self-esteem
- Sleeplessness
- Excessive talking
- Flight of ideas
- Distractibility
- Excessive goal-directed activity
- Excessive spending and buying sprees

A *depressive episode* is recognized by at least five of the following symptoms, persisting for at least two weeks, and one consisting of either depressed mood or loss of interest in activities:

- Depressed mood
- Loss of interest in activities
- Loss or abnormal increase in weight
- Inability to sleep or excessive sleepiness
- Restless or sluggish
- Excessive fatigue
- Guilt feelings
- Inability to think or concentrate
- Thoughts of death or suicide

Bipolar disorders are manic, depressive, or both, with recurring manic or depressive episodes, not necessarily meeting the full criteria for diagnosis.

Cyclothymia is characterized by hypomanic and depressed, but not major, episodes over one year or longer and never without some symptoms for more than two months at a time.

Dysthymia is a depressed or irritable mood occurring daily, without major depression, for at least one year and manifested by at least two of the following:

- Poor or excessive appetite
- Loss of or excess sleep
- Loss of energy or fatigue
- Poor self-esteem
- Inability to focus and concentrate
- Feelings of hopelessness

Anxiety Disorders

Anxiety disorders include panic disorder, phobias, obsessive compulsive disorder, post-traumatic stress disorder, and generalized anxiety disorder.

Panic disorders are characterized by shortness of breath, dizziness, rapid heart rate, trembling, sweating, and choking. Mitral valve prolapse may be associated with these symptoms, and amphetamine or caffeine toxicity, or elevated thyroid levels can mimic the syndrome.

Phobias include a fear of being alone in groups, in crowds, on bridges, and traveling alone (agoraphobia); and a fear of speaking in public or answering questions in class (social phobias). Children may have a fear of attending birthday parties or other group functions.

Obsessive compulsive disorder consists of recurrent and persistent, unreasonable ideas and thoughts (obsessions), and repetitive, purposeful, excessive behaviors in response to obsessions (compulsions). Examples of compulsive behavior include repetitive touching of objects and washing of hands.

Post-traumatic stress disorder is an abnormal reaction to a distressing event, characterized by recurring distressing recollections or dreams related to the trauma, avoidance of activities related to the trauma, sleep disturbance, irritability, and inability to concentrate on school work.

Generalized anxiety disorder consists of an abnormal degree of anxiety and worry about school grades and social interaction with peers. Symptoms include trembling, restlessness, palpitations, sweating, dizziness, difficulty concentrating, and irritability. Caffeine intoxication or excess thyroid can mimic the symptoms of anxiety disorder.

Prevalence of Psychiatric Disorders Among Children with ADHD

Children with ADHD complicated by severe mood disorders and anxiety disorders are likely to be referred primarily to the child psychiatrist or psychologist. Patients presenting with mild to moderate oppositional defiant and conduct disorders are often seen by the pediatrician and pediatric neurologist. Estimates of prevalence of comorbid disorders are dependent on the specialty of the treating physician; higher rates of occurrence might be expected among children referred to psychiatric clinics and psychologists. The majority of research studies involving ADHD children with comorbid psychiatric disorders have been conducted in psychiatry departments of major universities and medical centers. Lower prevalence rates might be expected among children treated in pediatric practice and child neurology clinics.

Relation Between Oppositional Defiant and Conduct Disorders and ADHD

Oppositional defiant disorder (ODD) comorbid with ADHD is a more common problem than conduct disorder (CD). The majority of children with ADHD do not have CD. Those who have CD develop the disorder before age 12 years, and almost always show symptoms of ODD for several years previously.

ODD children with CD, and those without, have different outcomes. CD with ADHD is associated with a higher frequency of substance abuse in adolescence, and higher incidence of anxiety and mood disorders.

The link between oppositional defiant disorder (ODD), conduct disorder (CD), and ADHD was evaluated at the *Pediatric Psychiatric Service, Massachusetts General Hospital, Boston* (Biederman et al., 1996):

- Of 140 children with ADHD, 65% had comorbid ODD and 22% had CD at initial examination.
- Of ODD children, 32% had comorbid CD.
- Children with CD also had ODD that preceded CD by several years.
- Children with both ODD and CD had more severe symptoms of ODD, more psychiatric disorders, including more bipolar disorder, and more abnormal behavior scores compared to ADHD children without comorbidity.

Neurological soft signs are found to correlate with the occurrence of symptoms of ODD and CD, as well as anxiety, phobias, depression or dysthymia. In a study of 56 high-risk boys, 7–10 years old, at the *New York State Psychiatric Institute, NY* (Pine et al., 1997), the demonstration of soft signs at neurological examination was a risk factor for childhood onset psychiatric symptoms, as well as ADHD.

Factors That Predispose to Conduct Disorders in Children with ADHD

ADHD and learning disabilities contribute to conduct disorders, but the main cause is linked to harsh, inconsistent parenting. Studies at *Queens College, Flushing, NY* (Halperin et al., 1997), and the *Institute of Psychiatry, London* (Scott, 1998), both demonstrated a relation between parent-aggressive behavior and aggression in the children, especially boys. Aggressive behavior occurred in 10% of children in an urban population, and the majority of juvenile delinquents had conduct disorders by age 7 years. Reduced serotonergic function, a neurochemical mechanism, was associated with aggression in the NY study.

Influence of an Adverse Family Environment on ADHD and Comorbid Disorders

Adverse family environments, chronic parental conflicts, and psychiatric illness affecting the mother influence the outcome of ADHD and the response to treatment. In a study of 140 ADHD children at the *Massachusetts General Hospital*, Biederman and associates (1995) found increased levels of environmental adversity among ADHD children compared to control subjects. Parental conflict and exposure to mothers with psychiatric illness were especially prevalent. Surprisingly, the risk of developing comorbid conduct disorder, depression, or anxiety was not influenced by environmental adverse factors.

In a study of psychiatric and developmental disorders in families of children with ADHD, researchers at the *University of Chicago* (Roizen et al., 1996) found that children with ADHD were more likely to have a parent affected by alcoholism, other drug abuse, depression, delinquency, learning disabilities, and/or ADHD. Children with a family history of psychiatric disorders should be screened for ADHD. Psychosocial intervention is recommended for families affected.

Childhood Conduct Disorder and Adult Criminality

Children with ADHD and conduct disorders are at increased risk for criminal behavior and arrest in adolescence and in adulthood (Satterfield and Schell, 1997). Childhood severe conduct disorders and adolescent antisocial behavior, if not treated by early psychosocial intervention, may be predictors of later arrest for criminality.

In some studies, hyperactive children are 5 times more likely to develop conduct disorders and a subsequent increased rate of criminality than average.

Relation of Mood and Anxiety Disorders to ADHD

Psychiatrists frequently find a cause and effect relationship between the symptoms of ADHD and anxiety or depression (Silver, 1992). In contrast, neurologists favor an organic biological etiology for ADHD and regard anxiety or mood disorders as secondary symptoms, sometimes precipitated by treatment (Millichap, 1997).

A depressive reaction induced by methylphenidate occurs particularly with larger doses and in children with a genetic vulnerability to mood disorders (Weinberg et al., 1997). Atomoxetine (Strattera®), a non-stimulant medication, may also be associated with mood disorder.

In a study at the *Massachusetts General Hospital, Boston,* a familial relationship between ADHD and bipolar disorder was examined in 140 affected children and their first-degree relatives (Faraone et al., 1997). The risk of bipolar disorder among relatives was increased fivefold if the child with ADHD also suffered from bipolar disorder. The comorbid presentation of ADHD and bipolar disorder appears to represent a distinct subtype of ADHD, predominantly affecting boys, and with a high familial risk of ADHD, bipolar disorder, and major depression. However, this subtype was rare, occurring in only 5% of children with ADHD. The findings did not support a theory of depression as a cause of ADHD.

Physicians are frequently faced with the differentiation of organic and psychiatric causes for behavioral and mood disorders complicated by complaints of hyperactivity, distractibility, and impulsivity. The recognition of early onset mood disorders should prompt withdrawal or dose reduction of stimulant or other therapy and referral to colleagues specializing in child psychology and psychiatry when appropriate.

Adolescent mania and ADHD. An association between adolescent mania and ADHD is reported from the Department of Psychiatry, *University of Cincinnati, Ohio* (West et al., 1995). Of 14 adolescent bipolar patients admitted to hospital for the treatment of acute mania or hypomania, 8 (57%) met the DSM criteria for a diagnosis of ADHD. Patients with ADHD had higher scores on a Mania Rating Scale than those with bipolar disorder alone.

Clinical symptoms and outcome of childhood-onset dysthymic disorder were compared with major depressive disorder in a 3- to 12-year study of two groups of school-age patients treated at the Psychiatric Departments of the *Universities of Pittsburgh, and California at San Diego,* and *Harvard University* (Kovacs et al., 1994). Dysthymic disorder had an earlier age of onset than major depressive disorder. Symptoms of feeling unloved, irritability and anger were similar, but guilt feelings, impaired concentration, loss of appetite, insomnia, and fatigue were less frequent than in major depression. Risk of major depressive disorder and bipolar disorder was increased in dysthymic patients.

Oppositional defiant and conduct disorders were present more often in a dysthymic group of patients than in those with major depression, treated as in-patients in a child psychiatry unit at *State University of New York at Stony Brook* (Ferro et al., 1994).

Children with the combined subtype of ADHD (inattentive and hyperactive-impulsive) showed the greatest psychiatric impairments compared to other subtypes in a study at the *Pediatric Psycho-pharmacology Unit, Massachusetts General Hospital, Boston* (Faraone et al., 1998). Hyperactive-impulsive patients were not different from controls on measures of depression, social functioning, IQ, and academic achievement.

ADHD and Drug Abuse Disorders in Adolescents

In an earlier study at the *Department of Psychiatry, Massachusetts General Hospital, Boston*, adolescents with ADHD had a similar risk of alcohol or drug abuse disorders as non-ADHD controls. At 4-year follow-up, drug abuse had occurred in 15% of 140 ADHD adolescents and with the same frequency in 120 normal control subjects. ADHD alone does not predispose to drug abuse during adolescence (Biederman et al., 1997). The risk of alcohol and drug abuse was increased in patients with a history of conduct or bipolar disorders, but not in those with oppositional defiant disorder, major depression, or anxiety. Oppositional defiant disorder, uncomplicated by conduct disorder, did not predispose to drug abuse.

Effect of Stimulant Treatment on Risk of Drug Abuse

Recent studies at *Massachusetts General Hospital* examined the effects of early stimulant medication for ADHD on the subsequent risk for substance use disorders (SUDs) and cigarette smoking in adolescent boys and girls. Stimulant-exposed adolescents with ADHD were 73% less likely to be diagnosed with SUD compared with those unexposed. Stimulant treatment for ADHD in childhood provides a significant protective effect on development of any SUD and cigarette smoking in adolescence ($P=0.001$). Risk of alcohol abuse or alcohol dependence is not affected by early stimulant treatment. (Biederman et al., 1999).

These reports should allay the common concern of parents whose child is prescribed stimulant medication for ADHD.

ADHD and Drug Abuse in Adults Compared to Adolescents

Studies show that adults with ADHD are more susceptible to drug abuse than adolescents. A sharp increase in drug abuse can be expected in adolescent ADHD subjects as they become adults, especially if they have not previously received treatment for ADHD.

Comorbid ADHD and substance abuse were studied in adolescents and adults at the *Veteran's Affairs Medical Center, West Haven, CT*. Substance use and abuse were related to attempts to self-medicate symptoms of ADHD, especially in previously untreated adolescents. Prescribed medical treatment for ADHD was found to decrease drug craving in adults with comorbid ADHD and drug abuse and to improve functioning (Horner and Scheibe, 1997).

Substance abuse disorder is commonly associated with a diagnosis of ADHD in adults. A study at the *Long Island Jewish Medical Center and NY State Psychiatric Institute* found that hyperactive boys with ADHD, when examined as adults, showed antisocial personality disorder and non-alcohol substance abuse in 12%, compared to 3% of controls (Mannuzza et al., 1998).

Biederman et al. (1995), at the *Massachusetts General Hospital,* found that childhood onset ADHD persisting in adults carried a 40% risk of substance abuse disorders, most commonly marijuana. The preferred drugs of abuse among adults with ADHD were not different from those used by normal control subjects. A concern of parents that ADHD children treated with methylphenidate may later show an increased tendency to abuse stimulant drugs was not supported.

Risk of ADHD Persistence into Adolescence

Risk factors for persistence of ADHD into adolescence include a genetic familial tendency to ADHD, psychosocial adversity and exposure to parental conflict, and comorbidity with conduct, mood and anxiety disorders (Biederman et al., 1995). Clearly, psychosocial intervention and appropriate medication at an early age are important in prevention of substance abuse disorders in adults with pervasive ADHD.

ADHD and Risk of Early Cigarette Smoking

ADHD is a significant risk factor for early cigarette smoking in children and adolescents, particularly when untreated or when associated with conduct disorder (Milberger et al., 1997). More recent studies at the *Massachusetts General Hospital, Boston*, show that children treated with stimulants have a 72% lower risk and later onset of cigarette smoking in adolescence (Wilens et al., 2008). Age at onset or duration of stimulant therapy had no effect on risk of cigarette smoking.

Neurological Basis for Obsessive Compulsive Disorder

Generally considered an anxiety neurosis, obsessive compulsive disorder (OCD) has recently been associated with structural abnormalities in the basal ganglia. In a study at the *Western Psychiatric Institute, University of Pittsburgh, PA*, MRI scans of 19 children, aged 7–18 years, with recent onset OCD showed significantly reduced volumes of the striatal basal ganglia (Rosenberg et al., 1997). Reduced striatal volume was correlated with the severity of OCD symptoms; the smaller the basal ganglia, the more severe the symptoms. These findings are in contrast to the acute enlargement of the basal ganglia that correlated with acute exacerbation of OCD and tics in a 12-year-old boy monitored by MRI at the *National Institute of Mental Health, Bethesda, MD* (Giedd et al., 1996). The symptoms followed a streptococcal throat infection, and treatment resulted in shrinkage in size of the basal ganglia and reduction in symptoms of OCD and tics. Structural changes in the brain correlating with severity of symptoms support an organic basis for OCD, but further and more definitive studies are indicated.

Other Comorbid Disorders Associated with ADHD

Developmental coordination disorder (Chap. 3), learning disabilities (Chap. 6), language delay (Chap. 6), tics, Tourette syndrome, seizure disorders, and headache (Chap. 7) are some of the disorders sometimes associated with ADHD. Their recognition and treatment are essential for the optimum management of ADHD. Sleep disturbance is considered a comorbid and causative factor by some researchers, whereas others discount a significant association with ADHD.

Asperger's Disorder (299.80) and ADHD

Asperger's syndrome is classified as a subgroup of autistic spectrum disorder (ASD) or pervasive developmental disorder (PDD). ADHD and Asperger's syndrome are often comorbid, despite the DSM-IV criteria for ADHD diagnosis that excludes PDD. Some children with ADHD may have an independent comorbid condition of PDD (Goldstein and Schwebach, 2004; Yoshida and Uchiyama, 2004). The DSM-IV criteria for Asperger's disorder (high-functioning ASD) are summarized as follows:

- Impairment in social interaction.
- Restricted repetitive and stereotyped patterns of behavior, interests, and activities.
- Significant impairments in social, occupational, or other areas of functioning.
- No delay in language development.
- No delay in cognitive development.
- No other pervasive developmental disorder.

The characteristic diagnostic criteria of Asperger's syndrome include a formal concrete way of thinking, and an inability to identify and understand human emotions and relationships. Communication difficulties range from stilted speech to almost robotic manner. Abnormal preoccupations include toy cars, insects, fungi, poisons, violence toward babies, ritualistic drawings, and excessive orderliness (Perkins and Wolkind, 1991; Tuchman, 1991). Asperger's syndrome may overlap or occur concurrently with Tourette syndrome (Nass and Gutman, 1997), and attention deficit disorder.

Symptoms that might be confused with ADHD are related to learning disorders, despite average or superior intelligence, especially areas involving language, spelling, reading, and visual memory. The neurological examination reveals motor incoordination and non-specific EEG abnormalities. A genetic factor is suspected but no specific organic pathology has been identified.

The manifestations of Asperger's syndrome that clearly distinguish this psychiatric disorder from ADHD are the peculiar personality and communication difficulties. Asperger's syndrome should be considered in children of high verbal intelligence who do poorly in school, both academically and socially, and who exhibit speech and language disorders, tics, motor clumsiness, and stereotyped movements such as repetitive hand flapping.

Multiple biological causes for autism and autistic-like disorders were uncovered in a study of 52 affected children examined neurologically at the *University of Goteborg, Sweden* (Steffenburg, 1991). The EEG was abnormal in 50% and the CT scan showed structural brain abnormalities in 25%.

The pediatric neurology examination is important in children with autistic-like symptoms, and EEG and CT/MRI may be indicated in selected patients. Biological disorders may be uncovered in children with symptoms thought to be primarily psychiatric and emotionally based (Millichap, 1994).

Sleep Disorders and ADHD

Sleep disorders sometimes associated with ADHD include restless legs syndrome/periodic limb movements, rhythmic movement disorder (body rocking and head banging), and parasomnias such as sleepwalking, sleep terrors, and confusional arousals. Increased associations are also reported between ADHD and hypersomnias such as narcolepsy and sleep apnea. Parents should be asked about sleep habits. (Walters et al., 2008).

Researchers *at University of North Carolina at Chapel Hill, Carrboro, NC,* examined the association between ADHD and parent-reported sleep problems among preschoolers aged 2–5 years. Of 1,073 parents who completed the Child Behavior Checklist, 193 children had high scores and 114 low scores. Neither hyperactive-impulsive nor inattentive ADHD symptoms were uniquely related to parent-reported problems involving sleep assistance, parasomnias, or dyssomnias. Inattentive symptomatology was related to daytime sleepiness. (Willoughby et al., 2008).

At *Penn State College of Medicine, Hershey, PA,* a study of 412 elementary schoolchildren, 6–12 years of age found that overnight polysomnograph sleep scores were not related to academic functioning. In contrast, IQ and neuropsychological test scores were powerful predictors of achievement. Children with and without sleep problems did not differ from each other in achievement, IQ, and ADHD symptoms. ADHD ratings were all significantly related to achievement (Mayes et al., 2008).

Summary

Psychiatric comorbidities associated with ADHD include oppositional defiant (ODD), conduct (CD), mood and anxiety disorders. ODD is especially prevalent in children with ADHD, occurring in 65% of patients referred to a Pediatric Psychiatric

Service; CD was found in 22% of cases. A lower incidence of psychiatric comorbidities is expected in pediatric or pediatric neurology clinics. Children with ADHD and CD are at increased risk for criminal behavior and arrest in adolescence and adulthood. Early psychosocial intervention is recommended. ADHD alone does not predispose to alcohol or drug abuse during adolescence, but the risk is increased in patients with comorbid CD or bipolar disorder. ODD uncomplicated by CD does not predispose to drug abuse. The evidence for a comorbid association of ADHD and sleep disorders is unconfirmed in some controlled studies.

Patients with ADHD treated early with stimulant medication are less likely to develop substance abuse disorders or to smoke cigarettes in adolescence. Childhood onset ADHD, untreated and persisting in adulthood, carries an increased risk of substance abuse disorders, most commonly marijuana, not stimulant medication. Risk factors for ADHD persistence in adolescence include a genetic familial tendency to ADHD, psychosocial adversity and exposure to parental conflict, and comorbidity with conduct, mood and anxiety disorders. Evidence for neurobiological causes of comorbid symptoms is provided by EEG and neuroimaging studies. Appropriate treatment of ADHD at an early age is important in prevention of substance abuse disorders in adolescence and pervasive ADHD in adulthood.

References

Biederman J, et al. Impact of adversity on functioning and comorbidity in children with attention-deficit hyperactivity disorder. *J Am Acad Child Adolesc Psychiatry*. 1995;34:1495–1503.

Biederman J, et al. Psychoactive substance use disorder in adults with attention deficit hyperactivity disorder (ADHD): effects of ADHD and comorbidity. *Am J Psychiatry*. 1995;152:1652–1658.

Biederman J, et al. Predictors of persistence and remission of ADHD into adolescence: results from a four-year prospective follow-up study. *J Am Acad Child Adolesc Psychiatry*. 1996;35: 343–351.

Biederman J, et al. Is childhood oppositional defiant disorder a precursor to adolescent conduct disorder? Findings from a four-year follow-up study of children with ADHD. *J Am Acad Child Adolesc Psychiatry*. 1996;35:1193–1204.

Biederman J, et al. Is ADHD a risk factor for psychoactive substance use disorders? Findings from a four-year prospective follow-up study. *J Am Acad Child Adolesc Psychiatry*. 1997;36:21–29.

Biederman J, Wilens TE, Mick E, Spencer T, Faraone SV. Pharmacotherapy of attention-deficit/hyperactivity disorder reduces risk for substance use disorder. *Pediatrics*. 1999;104:e20.

Faraone SV, et al. Attention-deficit hyperactivity disorder with bipolar disorder: a familial subtype? *J Am Acad Child Adolesc Psychiatry*. 1997;36:1378–1387.

Faraone SV, et al. Psychiatric, neuropsychological, and psychosocial features of DSM-IV subtypes of ADHD. *J Am Acad Child Adolesc Psychiatry*. 1998;37:185–193.

Ferro T, et al. Depressive disorders: Distinctions in children. *J Am Acad Child Adolesc Psychiatry*. 1994;33:664–670.

Giedd JN, et al. Case study: Acute basal ganglia enlargement and obsessive-compulsive symptoms in an adolescent boy. *J Am Acad Child Adolesc Psychiatry*. 1996;35:913–915.

Goldstein S, Schwebach AJ. The comorbidity of pervasive developmental disorder and attention deficit hyperactivity disorder: results of a retrospective chart review. *J Autism Dev Disord*. 2004;34:329–339.

Halperin JM, Newcom JH, Kopstein I, et al. Serotonin, aggression, and parental psychopathology in children with attention-deficit hyperactivity disorder. *J Am Acad Child Adolesc Psychiatry*. 1997;36:1391–1398.

Horner BR, Scheibe KE. Prevalence and implications of attention-deficit hyperactivity disorder among adolescents in treatment for substance abuse. *J Am Acad Child Adolesc Psychiatry*. 1997;36:30–36.

Kovacs M, et al. Childhood-onset dysthymic disorder. Clinical features and prospective naturalistic outcome. *Arch Gen Psychiatry*. 1994;51:365–374.

Mannuzza S, et al. Adult psychiatric status of hyperactive boys grown up. *Am J Psychiatry*. 1998;155:493–498.

Mayes SD, Calhoun SL, Bixler EO, Vgontzas AN. Nonsignificance of sleep relative to IQ and neuropsychological scores in predicting academic achievement. *J Dev Behav Pediatr*. 2008;29:206–212.

Milberger S, et al. ADHD is associated with early initiation of cigarette smoking in children and adolescents. *J Am Acad Child Adolesc Psychiatry*. 1997;36:37–44.

Millichap JG. *Progress in Pediatric Neurology II*. Chicago, IL: PNB Publishers; 1994.

Millichap JG. *Progress in Pediatric Neurology III*. Chicago, IL: PNB Publishers; 1997.

Nass R, Gutman R. Boys with Asperger's disorder, exceptional verbal intelligence, tics, and clumsiness. *Dev Med Child Neurol*. 1997;39:691–695.

Perkins M, Wolkind SN. Asperger's syndrome: who is being abused? *Arch Dis Child*. 1991;66:693–695.

Pine DS, et al. Neurological soft signs: one-year stability and relationship to psychiatric symptoms in boys. *J Am Acad Child Adolesc Psychiatry*. 1997;36:1579–1586.

Roizen NJ, et al. Psychiatric and developmental disorders in families of children with ADHD. *Arch Pediatr Adolesc Med*. 1996;150:203–208.

Rosenberg DR, et al. Frontostriatal measurement in treatment-naive children with obsessive-compulsive disorder. *Arch Gen Psychiatry*. 1997;54:824–830.

Satterfield JH, Schell A. A prospective study of hyperactive boys with conduct problems and normal boys: adolescent and adult criminality. *J Am Acad Child Adolesc Psychiatry*. 1997;36:1726–1735.

Scott S. Conduct disorder in children in the UK. *BMJ*. 1998;316:202–206.

Silver LB. *Attention-Deficit Hyperactivity Disorder. A Clinical Guide to Diagnosis and Treatment*. Washington, DC: American Psychiatric Press; 1992.

Steffenburg S. Neuropsychiatric assessment of children with autism: a population-based study. *Dev Med Child Neurol*. 1991;33:495–511.

Tuchman RF. Autism: delineating the spectrum. *Int Pediatr*. 1991;6:161–169.

Walters AS, Silvestri R, Zucconi M, Chandrashekariah R, Konofal E. Review of the possible relationship and hypothetical links between attention deficit hyperactivity disorder (ADHD) and the simple sleep related movement disorders, parasomnias, hypersomnias, and circadian rhythm disorders. *J Clin Sleep Med*. 2008;4:591–600.

Weinberg WA, et al. Depressive reaction induced by methylphenidate. *J Pediatr*. 1997;130:665–669.

West SA, et al. ADHD and adolescent mania. *Am J Psychiatry*. 1995;152:271–273.

Willoughby MT, Angold A, Egger HL. Parent-reported attention-deficit/hyperactivity disorder symptomatology and sleep problems in a preschool-age pediatric clinic sample. *J Am Acad Child Adolesc Psychiatry*. 2008;47:1086–1094.

Yoshida Y, Uchiyama T. The clinical necessity for assessing attention deficit/hyperactivity disorder (AD/HD) symptoms in children with high-functioning pervasive developmental disorder (PDD). *Eur Child Adolesc Psychiatry*. 2004;13:307–314.

Chapter 6
Learning and Language Disorders

Learning and language disorders frequently complicate attention deficit disorder, and their recognition and remediation are essential for the successful management of ADHD. Specific learning disorders that involve the "three Rs" are termed dyslexia, dysgraphia, and dyscalculia. Dyslexia or reading disability is the prototype of learning disabilities. Speech and language disorders include dysarthrias, or disorders of articulation, and aphasias or dysphasias, inabilities to comprehend and use language despite normal hearing and intellect.

Of 119 children, ages 8–16 years, evaluated in a child diagnostic clinic at *Department of Psychiatry, Penn State University College of Medicine,* a learning disability (LD) was present in 70% of children with ADHD. LD in written expression was two times more common (65%) than an LD in reading, math, or spelling. Children with LD and ADHD had more severe learning problems than children who had LD but no ADHD. LD and attention problems are on a continuum, are interrelated, and usually coexist (Mayes et al., 2000).

Comorbidity with LD is a modifying factor in the health-related quality of life of children with ADHD. At the *University of British Columbia, Canada,* a questionnaire survey of 131 families of children diagnosed with ADHD found 51(39%) with comorbid learning disorder, and 45(34%) having oppositional defiant disorder or conduct disorder (Klassen et al., 2004). Estimates of the prevalence of ADHD and learning disability (LD) in US children 6–17 years of age, 2004–2006, at the *National Center for Health Statistics, Hyattsville, MD,* found 5% of children had ADHD without LD, 5% had LD without ADHD, and 4% had both ADHD and LD. Boys were more likely than girls to have each of the diagnoses (Pastor and Reuben, 2008).

Neurological assessment is recommended in children with learning disabilities who fail to show academic progress despite appropriate educational intervention. At *the Neuropediatric Unit, Shaare Zedek Medical Center, Jerusalem, Israel,* 7 third-grade children with developmental dyscalculia had neurological disorders with direct bearing on the cognitive disabilities and remedial therapy (Shalev and Gross-Tsur, 1993). Four had ADHD, one had absence seizures, one had dyslexia for numbers, and another had Gerstmann syndrome, a parietal lobe disorder resulting in LD affecting handwriting and arithmetic.

J.G. Millichap, *Attention Deficit Hyperactivity Disorder Handbook,*   59
DOI 10.1007/978-1-4419-1397-5_6, © Springer Science+Business Media, LLC 2010

A sample of 235 families with ADHD was assessed for familial association with LD at the *University of California, Los Angeles.* The prevalence rates were highest for reading disability, followed by writing (dysgraphia), then math disability (dyscalculia). Strong familial association was demonstrated for reading disability, with weaker association for writing disability. Independent familial factors appeared to underlie ADHD and LD (Del'Homme et al., 2007).

Definitions of Dyslexia

Dyslexia is a disorder manifested by a difficulty in learning to read despite conventional instruction, adequate intelligence, and socio-cultural opportunity. It is dependent on fundamental cognitive disabilities that are frequently of constitutional origin (World Federation of Neurology definition, Waites, 1968).

More current definitions, accepted by the International Dyslexia Association, include the following: *Dyslexia* is a neurologically-based, often familial, disorder, which interferes with the acquisition and processing of language. *Dyslexia* is one of several distinct learning disabilities. Dyslexia is a specific language-based disorder of constitutional origin characterized by difficulties in single word decoding that reflect insufficient phonological processing.

Earlier suggestions that dyslexia is due to an immaturity of cerebral function are supported by MRI evidence of developmental cerebral anomalies (Galaburda et al., 1985). The anatomical location of these anomalies correlates with a "phonological-linguistic," or deficient speech sound and decoding basis for dyslexia (Denckla, 1994). An alternative theory, now less accepted, proposed a defect in the visual system and perception of letters and words. Some authorities regard reading ability and disability as a continuum, with differences in degree but not in kind (Shaywitz et al., 1995).

The left temporal-parietal area appears to be most critical in the anatomical localization of normal reading ability, but additional areas of the left hemisphere may be involved also. Some reports of acquired dyslexia following surgery on the brain have involved the left frontal lobe. A *disconnection theory* involving impaired relays between the anterior and posterior areas of the left brain has been proposed.

Dyslexia occurs in 5–10% of school children, at all levels of intelligence, from superior to low normal. Dyslexia may be an isolated abnormality or may be associated with other learning disabilities. Reading and spelling disability overlaps with ADHD and shows similar genetic characteristics but different brain localizations. Anatomically, left hemisphere deficits are associated with reading and other learning disabilities, whereas the right frontal lobe is involved in ADHD. Attentional mechanisms affected in children with ADHD are considered an important underlying factor in developmental dyslexia. Pharmacological treatment for ADHD offers a potential adjunct to teaching dyslexic readers to read fluently and automatically (Shaywitz and Shaywitz, 2008).

Early Signs of Dyslexia

The dyslexic child is able to learn simple words by rote memory or by association with pictures or other cues but makes frequent errors in pronunciation and often substitutes words of similar meanings. The most frequent signs of dyslexia are as follows:

- Failure to distinguish mirror-image letters, "d" and "b" and the words "big" and "dig."
- Reversal of letters, e.g., "was" for "saw."
- Substitutions, e.g., "bed" for "bad."
- Omissions, e.g., "soon" for "spoon."
- Extra phonemes, e.g., "open" for "pen."

The reading level is determined by standard tests such as the Jastak test of word recognition and pronunciation and Gray's oral reading paragraphs.

The Genetic Factor in Reading Disability

The strong predilection for boys is well-documented but the method of genetic transmission of dyslexia is less well defined. Nancy Millichap, in her thesis on dyslexia (1986), reviewed studies of twins and found evidence in support of a genetic influence. Of a total of 96 twin pairs reported in the literature, 36 (88%) monozygotic twins were concordant for dyslexia compared to only 16 (29%) dizygotic twins. Between 25 and 50% of children with reading disability show a hereditary influence, with autosomal dominant, sex-linked recessive, and polygenetic transmission. The genetic pattern depends in part on the definition and the association with other learning disabilities in the families studied.

A subsequent twin study at the *Hospital for Sick Children, London, UK*, showed that genetic factors play a moderate role in reading retardation and a stronger influence in spelling disability (Stevenson et al., 1987). A twin study at the *University of New South Wales, Australia*, involved children with ADHD complicated by reading and speech problems. Male twins were affected more frequently than female, and the reading disability in male twins became more severe in adolescence while that in female twins showed improvement (Levy et al., 1996).

ADHD and reading disability tend to co-occur, and molecular genetic studies support the hypothesis that the alpha 2A adrenergic receptor (ADRAZA) gene is contributing to this association (Stevenson et al., 2005). Linkage and association studies in dyslexia suggest that a susceptibility locus exists on chromosome 15q15-q21 (Schumacher et al., 2008). Further systematic studies are required to identify the true dyslexia susceptibility gene(s).

Evidence for a Neuroanatomical Basis for Dyslexia

Neuroanatomical and related studies in dyslexics have led to a so-called neural signature of dyslexia (Shaywitz and Shaywitz, 2008). Since the original *Harvard University* study showing cerebral developmental anomalies in CT scans of four dyslexic male subjects (Galaburda et al., 1985), the findings have been confirmed at autopsy in three women with dyslexia. Microscopic scars in the brains were linked to lupus erythematosus in the mother, and an immune mechanism for dyslexia was proposed (Humphreys et al., 1990). Left-handedness was more important than immune disorders in a study of associated factors in dyslexic children at the *Center for Reading Research, Stavanger, Norway* (Tonnessen et al., 1993).

A reappraisal of the anatomical basis for dyslexia using MRI studies at *Yale University School of Medicine, New Haven, CT*, concluded that differences in sex, age, handedness, and the definition of dyslexia could explain discrepancies in brain region volumes in children with dyslexia and other learning disabilities (Schultz et al., 1994). A small corpus callosum was a further cerebral anomaly discovered in MRI studies of dyslexic children at the *University of Georgia, Augusta* (Hynd et al., 1995). Familial left-handedness and ADHD distinguished the dyslexic children from control children in the study. Measurements of the corpus callosum in genetic studies of twin pairs at *Dartmouth Medical School* (1989) showed greater conformity and might be more reliable in anatomical dyslexic studies (Millichap, 1997).

MRI and CT measurements of brain regions in dyslexic subjects have provided evidence of anomalies suggesting interruptions in brain development, possibly related to immune mechanisms. These studies are investigational and the anomalies are insufficiently documented for use in diagnosis.

In addition to studies of the neuroanatomy of developmental dyslexia in subjects born with the disorder, occasional cases are described in adults with acquired dyslexia who have undergone surgery for cerebral tumor or other discretely localized brain lesions. A right-handed woman, a patient at the *University of Iowa College of Medicine*, developed severe dyslexia and dysgraphia following the surgical removal of a small tumor located in the left premotor frontal lobe. By contrast, she was able to write numbers and perform written calculations without difficulty. The isolated simultaneous occurrence of dyslexia and dysgraphia, without dyscalculia, is rare. This case report suggests that the frontal lobe of the brain may be involved in some cases of dyslexia (Anderson et al., 1990). Figure 6.1 shows the anatomy of language and areas of representation of dyslexia, dysgraphia, dyscalculia, and dysphasia.

Brain Imaging Scanners Used in Dyslexia Research

The *PET (Positron-emission tomography)* scanner, developed in 1974, provides images of brain metabolic activity using radioactive tracer isotopes. Radiologists using PET scanners inject water containing the isotope oxygen-15 into the blood-stream, and the positrons emitted by the isotope produce energy that is picked up by radiation detectors on the scalp. The resulting images are color coded by computers and reflect areas of increased blood flow. The *fMRI (Functional magnetic resonance imaging)*, a more sensitive scanner than PET, also relies on an increase in cerebral blood flow to show changes in brain cell activity in various locations. Both these machines demonstrate regional changes within seconds whereas nerve cells transmit messages in milliseconds. Neither the PET nor the fMRI will determine the order and timing of processes involved in the recognition of letters and words.

Magnetoencephalography (MEG) is employed to track noninvasively in milliseconds the brain activation sequences during reading. The EEG detects electrical currents in the brain, while the MEG promptly records the magnetic effects of these currents. The fMRI can be used for localization of the brain activity during reading and MEG for the timing of the process, a spatial-temporal measuring device, or magnetic source imaging.

Brain Activation During Reading

Magnetic source imaging (MSI), a combination of magnetoencephalography (MEG) and the anatomic images on MRI, has been used to provide anatomic location of brain activity at a given time, during reading by dyslexics and normal readers. In a study at the *University of Helsinki, Finland*, dyslexics failed to activate the left visual and receptive language cortical areas during word presentation, but instead, activated the left inferior frontal lobe (Salmelin et al., 1996).

An impaired perception of visual word processing of written words resulted from a dysfunction of auditory language areas in the left temporal lobe. The activation of the left posterior temporal lobe during reading aloud or silently has been observed in PET studies of normal readers examined at the *Hammersmith Hospital, London* (Price et al., 1994). The most critical neuroanatomical area of dysfunction in dyslexic subjects is the left posterior temporal, a region of the brain that governs the understanding of spoken words and also transmits visual perception fiber tracts.

More recent functional neuroimaging studies at *Stanford University, Palo Alto, CA*, confirm previous reports and show that adults and children with developmental dyslexia exhibit reduced parietotemporal activation (Hoeft et al., 2006). To determine more specific neural correlates of dyslexia, these investigators conducted a functional MRI study with a rhyme judgment task, comparing reading ability and scanner performance in dyslexic children and normal readers. Dyslexic children exhibited reduced activation in the left parietotemporal cortex and five other regions, including the right parietotemporal cortex. Activation differences seen in dyslexic children were unrelated to either current reading level or scanner task performance, but instead represented an atypical developmental neural system.

Widespread activation across the cerebellar hemispheres, in addition to cerebral activation, is reported in an fMRI study using a noun–verb association paradigm at the *University of Brussels, Belgium* (Baillieux et al., 2008). A new hypothesis for the pathophysiological mechanisms of developmental dyslexia is proposed that involves the processing or transfer of information within the cerebellar cortex.

Evidence for a Visual Pathway Disorder in Dyslexics

A number of highly sophisticated studies including visual evoked potentials have pointed to deficits in the visualization of letters and whole words in some dyslexics. Scientists from the *Research Laboratory of Electronics* and the *Departments of Biology, Electrical Engineering and Computer Science at MIT, Cambridge, MA,* have collaborated in an investigation of the peripheral and central vision of 5 dyslexic adult subjects compared to 5 normal readers. Dyslexics have impairments of letter discrimination in the central field of vision and better than normal peripheral vision for letter identification. After a program of exercises involving spatial organization and eye–hand coordination and the use of a device to utilize peripheral vision in reading, the recognition of letters by severe dyslexics was significantly improved. Dyslexics should be taught to read using peripheral vision (Geiger and Lettvin, 1987).

Slowing of visual evoked responses in reading-disabled children has been demonstrated at the *School of Optometry, University of Missouri, St Louis* (Lehmkuhle et al., 1993). MEG and MRI studies also point to involvement of cerebral visual pathways and function as well as receptive language centers. Although a so-called "phonolinguistic" theory of dyslexia (inability to recognize and decode speech sounds or phonemes) is favored, deficits in the visualization of words appear to be important in some dyslexic subjects. These two types of dyslexia have been termed *dysphonetic and dyseidetic* (Boder, 1973). Dysphonetic dyslexics compensate by becoming visual spellers, while dyseidetic dyslexics use auditory pathways and phonics. A multisensory approach to remedial reading is recommended for hyperactive children with ADD complicated by reading disability.

Articulatory Feedback and Disconnection Theories of Dyslexia

Researchers at the *University of Florida, Gainesville*, FL, have proposed a motor-articulatory feedback hypothesis to explain developmental dyslexia (Heilman et al., 1996). The authors theorize that most children learn to read by the alphabetic system, requiring speech sound (phonological) awareness and conversion of letters (graphemes) into speech sounds (phonemes). Most dyslexics have deficient phonological awareness and difficulty converting graphemes into phonemes. The left inferior frontal lobe, involved in articulation, is important in phonological reading, as demonstrated in PET studies. Dyslexic children are unable to perceive the position and movement of the articulatory muscles (mouth, lips, tongue) during speech. Their phonological awareness and ability to convert graphemes to phonemes is impaired. Deficits in programming or feedback of motor articulation are related to this lack of awareness of the muscles of articulation.

A *disconnection* theory involving impaired relays between anterior and posterior language areas of the brain is proposed by investigators at the *MRC Cognitive Development Unit, London, UK* (Paulesu et al., 1996). Using PET to study brain activity in 5 adults with developmental dyslexia, left hemisphere brain regions normally activated in phonological processing were defective.

Selection of Reading Remediation Methods for Dyslexics

Subtyping of dyslexic children proposed by Boder (1973) is validated by neurophysiological tests and may be used in the choice of remediation methods (Flynn and Deering, 1989). In a study at the *Gunderson Clinic, LaCrosse, WI*, dyslexic subgroups, *dysphonetic* (with auditory-phonetic disabilities), and *dyseidetic* (visual-spatial disabilities), showed significant differences on tests of reading and in EEG activity over the left temporal-parietal, angular gyrus, an area involved in phonetic decoding. This area showed overuse or increased activity in the dyseidetic children who audibly decoded words, whereas dysphonetic dyslexics skipped unknown words or substituted words with the same beginning sound.

The Boder test is based on the premise that dyslexic readers have characteristic patterns of strengths and weaknesses in two distinct cognitive components of the reading process: (1) the visual gestalt function and (2) the auditory analytic function. The visual gestalt function underlies the ability to develop a sight vocabulary. The auditory analytic function governs phonic word-analysis skills. These two cognitive functions are basic to the two standard methods of initial reading instruction: (1) the whole word method and (2) the phonic method. The Boder test results are helpful to the educator in the choice of remediation methods. The matching method or *neuropsychological approach* to reading remediation involves matching the learning strengths with a teaching strategy designed to exploit these strengths. This matching method appears to be theoretically sound and much preferred to techniques based on deficit remediation, involving the training or retraining of damaged or dysfunctional areas of the brain.

Alternative Methods of Reading Remediation

A wide variety of methods of reading remediation have been recommended, beginning with the multisensory (phonetic-kinesthetic) technique described by Orton (1937), Gillingham and Stillman (1940), Fernald (1943), and Strauss and Lehtinen (1947). An excellent review of these and other methods of reading remediation is provided by Millichap (1986).

The *multisensory method* is included in the category known as the *one best method* or *VAKT*, which stands for visual, auditory, kinesthetic, and tactile stimulation. In learning a word by the VAKT approach, the child sees the word, hears the teacher say the word, and simultaneously says the word, traces it, and feels the muscle movement and touch sensation in the fingers.

Critics of the multisensory approach are concerned about the rigidity of the teaching method, the tendency to belabor reading, and the lack of emphasis on comprehension. The emphasis on phonics precludes its application with dysphonetic dyslexic children or those weak in auditory perception.

Deficit remediation method is a category of remedial reading focused on remediation of prerequisite reading readiness skills that are presumed lacking in the dyslexic child. Proponents (Kephart, Frostig, Doman-Delacato, and Kirk) theorized that perceptual motor, cerebral dominance, and psycholinguistic skills must be developed as a foundation for reading readiness. Critics argue that the treatment methods lack proof of effectiveness, and techniques based on deficit remediation may lead to poor self-concept and negative attitudes toward reading and school in general (Hynd and Cohen, 1983; Hartlage, 1981).

Alternatives to the deficit remediation methods are those that determine each child's intact areas of neurological functioning and match cognitive neuropsychological strengths with a teaching strategy designed to exploit these strengths. This matching method is sometimes termed the *neuropsychological approach* to reading remediation and is favored by experts including Johnson and Myklebust, Boder, and Mattis. A battery of psychological tests to assess the child's cognitive abilities is a prerequisite to the choice of method of reading remediation. Those with stronger phono-linguistic abilities are taught by the phonic and decoding methods, and those with weak phonic abilities and normal visual-spatial function may respond better to a look-say, whole-word or a multisensory approach.

Audiovisual training is an effective method of remediation, recently demonstrated in 23 children with dyslexia and 23 control average readers studied at *University of Lyon, France* (Veuillet et al., 2007). Impairment of auditory processing skills was measured using a categorical perception task that assesses the processing of a phonemic contrast based on voice onset time (VOT) and medial olivocochlear (MOC) function. VOT refers to the time between onset of voice (laryngeal vibration) and its release from mouth closure. Audiovisual training significantly improved reading and voicing sensitivity.

Dyslexics have a sensory temporal processing deficit that impairs the ability to relate word sounds and letter sounds and to associate the printed letter (grapheme) with the appropriate speech sound (phoneme). Audiovisual training reverses the deficient phonological awareness and facilitates conversion of graphemes to phonemes (Magnan et al., 2004; Merzenich et al., 1996).

Computer-Based Language Exercises

Computer-based intervention targeting auditory temporal processing combined with language exercises (Fast ForWord R) failed to benefit children with impairments in reading, phonemic awareness, spelling, and language skills (Given et al., 2008). In contrast, reading and written language improvements in passage comprehension and spelling are reported following treatment of a dyslexic child using Fast ForWord exercises, when demonstrated by magnetoencephalography (Lajiness-O'Neill et al.,

2007). Further investigation of computer-based training with ortho-phonological units in dyslexic children may be indicated (Ecalle et al., 2008).

Dietary and Pharmacological Therapies

Dietary supplementation with long-chain polyunsaturated fatty acids, omega-3 and omega-6, is the latest alternative, complementary treatment proposed in the management of dyslexia in children. Fatty acid deficiencies reported in children with ADHD and dyslexia may be involved in the associated impairments of dopaminergic cortico-striatal metabolism. Although responses are mixed, some controlled studies have demonstrated significant improvements in reading, spelling, and ADHD behavior over 3 months trial of fatty acids (Richardson and Montgomery, 2005; Richardon, 2006; Frolich and Dopfner, 2008). A more recent study failed to confirm the hypothesis that omega-3 fatty acid (ethyl-eicosapentaenoic acid, EPA) or carnosine has a role in the treatment of reading and spelling problems in children with dyslexia (Kairaluoma et al., 2008). Different populations and forms of fatty acid may explain the contrasting results of these trials. The patients attending our ADD Clinic in Chicago who have supplemented stimulant treatment with fish oil capsules report mixed benefits in behavior or reading proficiency. Reading disability associated with ADHD may benefit from stimulant therapy and improvement in attention.

Prognosis of Developmental Dyslexia

Dyslexic children often come to the remedial setting after several years of frustration due to poor academic success in the regular classroom. The child's self-concept is low, and he/she may have a comorbid attention deficit hyperactivity disorder. A reconditioning period is often advisable, during which behavior modification is employed along with medications to improve attention.

Under favorable conditions most dyslexic children can be taught to read by appropriate remedial methods, but a minority of severely disabled children remain illiterate despite all efforts made by qualified tutors. The ability to read should not be confused with intelligence, and poor readers are not necessarily poor learners. Indeed, some dyslexic children have entered professions and have enjoyed success in adult life by compensating for their disability. The relative importance of reading in learning may need to be de-emphasized and alternative channels such as audiovisual materials employed to teach children with severe dyslexia refractory to therapy. Case histories of dyslexic children are provided in Millichap and Millichap (1986).

Writing and Arithmetic Learning Disorders

Dysgraphia, or agraphia, is an inability to write or print words and numbers in the absence of paralysis of the arm or hand. It is essentially an apraxia involving the hand. Mild cases may be manifested by contraction of words, elision of letters or

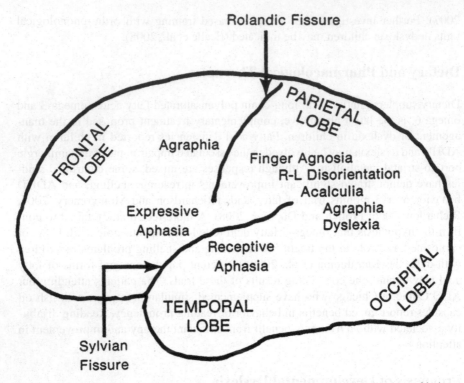

Fig. 6.1 Diagram of left cerebral hemisphere showing the neuroanatomic localizations of lesions causing disorders of language and learning

syllables, poor spacing of letters and words, or mirror writing. Dysgraphia often complicates aphasia and dyslexia. Anatomically, the hand area or Exner's writing center is located in the middle frontal convolution of the left frontal lobe. Dysgraphia may also follow a posterior cerebral lesion and may be part of the Gerstmann syndrome (Fig. 6.1).

Gerstmann syndrome consists of the following disabilities, as shown in Fig. 6.1:

- *Finger agnosia,* or an inability to recognize, name, or select individual fingers of the hand.
- *Right-left disorientation,* or confused laterality.
- *Agraphia,* or an inability to write.
- *Acalculia,* an inability to count or to understand arithmetical problems.

Gerstmann syndrome is described in adults with tumors and stroke lesions involving the angular gyrus, in the temporo-parietal cortex of the dominant hemisphere. Partial syndromes may occur with localized lesions of other cerebral cortical regions or even with diffuse cerebral pathology. Gerstmann syndrome occurs in children with ADHD who have learning disorders affecting handwriting and arithmetic.

Dyscalculia is an inability to learn arithmetic and do simple arithmetical calculations. A child's development of numerical concepts begins as early as one year of age with his manipulation of one object after another. As a prerequisite to counting he gains insight into concepts of size, number, and form by playing with form boards, puzzles, and boxes. He learns about sequence and order by stringing beads or putting pegs in boards, and he adds to his ideas of quantity by learning phrases such as "all gone," "no more," and "too much."

Mathematical concepts include receptive and expressive aspects just as other forms of symbolic language, and modern methods of teaching mathematics emphasize meaning rather than rote learning. A child with dyscalculia is unable to understand mathematical principles and processes, but in addition, he may have difficulty re-visualizing numbers, writing numbers, or understanding and remembering instructions. An auditory receptive language disorder will not affect arithmetical computation, but math involving reasoning and vocabulary will be weakened. Deficits in auditory memory and recall of numbers interfere with a child's mathematical performance because he cannot listen and assimilate all of the facts presented orally. Oral work should be minimized when auditory memory is impaired.

Dyslexia and visual perceptual disturbances resulting in confusion of letters may interfere with the ability to read and understand mathematical problems but do not impair calculation when problems are read aloud. Dyslexic children have little difficulty in learning arithmetic when presented with numerical symbols, but they are unable to solve problems in which the written word is used instead.

Children with dysgraphia may have difficulty in writing numerals as well as words. The use of problems with multiple-choice answers that can be encircled or underlined will prevent arithmetical failure due to apraxic disorders.

At the Schneider Children's Medical Center, Jerusalem, Israel, an 11 year-old, Hebrew-speaking boy of normal intelligence was referred for evaluation of learning and attentional problems and was found to have a profound dyscalculia based on a proposed lack of "cardinal/ordinal skills acquisition device" (COSAD). Several male family members had dysgraphia, right-left disorientation, and dyslexia. At birth, the child was hypotonic, and motor development was delayed, walking independently at 2 and 1/2 years.

Neurological abnormalities included high-pitched voice, dysgraphia, right-left disorientation, finger agnosia, clumsiness in running and jumping, scoliosis, and fine motor incoordination. At 4 years, he developed grand mal seizures treated with carbamazepine, and at 7 years he received pemoline (Cylert) for ADD without hyperactivity. The pemoline benefited overall functioning. The use of linguistic, visual, and verbal memory cues compensated for deficits in ordinal number use, but not for cardinal number skills, which remained limited. He could count small numbers, but could not do simple calculations, a skill requiring an innate experience of quantity, less amenable to language, visuo-spatial, or logical mediation (Ta'ir et al., 1997).

Profound developmental dyscalculia and Gerstmann's syndrome may occur in children of normal or even superior intelligence. Deficits in specific cognitive areas may involve visuo-spatial perception and parietal-occipital dysfunction. In a theoretical hypothesis of developmental dyscalculia, an innate, highly specific cognitive domain is involved. Ordinal number tasks and counting small magnitudes may be successfully completed, whereas larger quantities involving calculations are not possible.

Influence of Gender on Attention and Learning Ability

Girls with ADHD have a relatively greater tendency to be inattentive than hyperactive-impulsive, whereas neuropsychological deficits involving executive function, the ability to organize and monitor thoughts and behavior, are less remarkable in girls than in boys. Compared to normal controls, girls with ADHD are significantly more impaired on tests of attention, intellectual performance, and achievement, and have higher rates of learning disability. However, impairments of cognitive function, attention, arithmetic, and reading are common to both sexes affected by ADHD (Seidman et al., 1997).

Speech and Language Disorders

Normal Development of Speech and Language

An infant says the first intelligible word by about 1 year of age. During the second year the child recognizes the names of familiar objects and parts of the body and begins to form short phrases. In the third year he uses speech for toilet needs and social interaction in play, and at 4 years he can repeat songs and nursery rhymes. A useful index of a child's development of language is the length of the response when presented with a familiar picture or toy: the response is 2 words at 2 years of age, 4 words at 3 years, 6 words at 5 years, and 8 words at 8 years.

Signs of Language Delay

A delay in saying the first word beyond 18 months may indicate a physical, mental, or hearing disability. Hearing should be checked in early infancy, especially if the child suffers from repeated ear infections or a family member has a hearing problem.

Failure to put 2 or 3 words together in short phrases by 2 years and sentences by the age of 3 years is a sign of significant language delay.

Dysarthria is a disability involving the neuromuscular control of speech and articulation. *Aphasia* or *dysphasia* is a failure or impairment of the understanding or use of language in the absence of deafness or mental retardation.

Types of Aphasia and Their Treatment

Congenital aphasia (or dysphasia) is a developmental language deficit that is recognized in the first year or two of life. *Acquired aphasia* presents after the acquisition of language has begun, and results from lesions in the language areas of the brain.

Aphasia acquired by children is usually reversible if the cause is localized and nonprogressive, as with trauma related lesions. The opposite hemisphere of the brain assumes the function of the dominant side. In adults, acquired aphasia is either permanent or resolves slowly and incompletely in response to therapy. Childhood aphasia due to infection, vascular disease, or that associated with epilepsy has a poor outcome (Loonen and van Dongen, 1990). *Epileptic aphasia*, or Landau-Kleffner syndrome, is an acquired form of aphasia that affects children with epilepsy and develops between 2 and 5 years of age.

Aphasias are also classified as *expressive, receptive,* or *expressive-receptive.* Expressive aphasia is an apraxia, or loss of purposeful movements of the muscles of speech or writing in the absence of paralysis. Receptive aphasia is a visual and auditory agnosia, or inability to interpret or comprehend the significance of written or spoken words despite normal vision and hearing. In *amnesic* or *nominal* aphasia the child has difficulty in finding the name of an object while understanding its purpose and correct usage (Nielsen, 1965).

The differentiation of aphasia from mental retardation or infantile autism may be difficult, but the aphasic child's general performance and facial expressive communication are more adequately developed and well in advance of language performance.

Six syndromes of developmental dysphasia and their remediation were identified at the International Child Neurology Congress held in Jerusalem, Israel, 1986. The differentiation of subtypes of developmental and acquired dysphasias in young children is facilitated by the MRI, which sometimes uncovers subtle cerebral anomalies. Some syndromes result from genetic neurodevelopmental abnormalities while other dysphasias are caused by acquired lesions, before or at birth. Early therapeutic intervention may stimulate brain reorganization and development of alternative pathways (Allen et al., 1989).

Prognosis of developmental aphasia. The language growth in 26 two-year old children with expressive language delay was studied at the *State University of New York, Stony Brook, NY* (Fischel et al., 1989). After a 5-month follow-up period, improvement was variable, with 1/3 showing no improvement, 1/3 mild improvement, and 1/3 having normal language development. Predictors of improvement included the child's 2-year vocabulary size used at home, regular meal times, and the extent of quiet interaction between mother and child. The effectiveness of early intervention programs for language development outside the home was generally disappointing. More accurate diagnosis of subtypes of dysphasia might lead to more specific intervention techniques with more effective results.

Developmental dysphasia may be complicated by ADHD, adding to the problems of treatment.

A 7-year-old girl with developmental dysphasia, examined at the *Medical College of Georgia, Augusta, GA*, was treated with methylphenidate for ADHD. She had said her first words late at 2 years and short phrases at 4 years of age. Her 6-year-old brother had developmental dyslexia of the dysphonetic type. Speech and language evaluations at 3 years of age showed no expressive language; the child communicated her wishes by pointing and gesturing. Receptive language was at an 18-month level, and play audiometry revealed normal hearing. Her intelligence level was 70. In contrast to weaknesses in language and vocabulary development, her visual-spatial perception and construction abilities were relatively strong. A neurodevelopmental anomaly affecting the left frontal cortex was diagnosed, and a genetic basis for the language delay was suggested by the family history of learning disability (Cohen et al., 1989).

Methods of Treatment of Aphasia

Researchers at *Rutgers University, Newark, NJ*, and *University of California, San Francisco, CA* report an exciting new method for the treatment of dysphasia that uses acoustically-modified synthetic speech (Tallal et al., 1996). Deficits in recognition and processing of rapidly successive phonetic elements of speech in language-impaired children, aged 5–10 years, were improved by listening to synthetic speech. The acoustically-modified speech is presented at a slower rate on audiotapes and by daily training with computer games designed to modify phoneme perception. After 1 month of daily training exercises, test scores improved by 2 years, and normal levels of speech discrimination and language comprehension were achieved. Compared to a control group of language-learning impaired children receiving natural speech training, those treated with acoustically modified speech training showed significantly larger improvements. If confirmed, this method of language training intervention will improve the outcome of developmental dysphasia.

Summary

The recognition and remediation of associated learning and language disabilities are important for the successful management of ADHD. Learning disability (LD) is a frequent comorbidity, estimated to occur in 39–70% of children with ADHD. LD and attention problems are on a continuum, are interrelated, and generally coexist. Neurological assessment is recommended in children with LD who fail to make academic progress despite appropriate educational intervention. The prevalence rate for various LD is highest for reading disability, followed by writing and math disabilities. Dyslexia occurs in 5–10% of school children; it overlaps with ADHD and shows similar genetic characteristics but different brain localizations. Anatomically, left hemisphere deficits are associated with reading and other LD, whereas the right frontal lobe is involved in ADHD. Attentional mechanisms affected in children with ADHD are also important in developmental dyslexia.

Writing (agraphia) and math (acalculia) disabilities, in association with finger agnosia and right–left disorientation, occur as the Gerstmann syndrome in adults with tumor or stroke involving the angular gyrus of the dominant hemisphere. The syndrome, often in a partial form, may be found in children with ADHD and LD affecting handwriting and arithmetic. Language delays, receptive and expressive, may also complicate ADHD and LD, impacting the response to remedial therapy.

References

Allen DA, Mendelson L, Rapin I. Syndrome specific remediation in preschool developmental dysphasia. In French JH et al. eds. *Child Neurol and Dev Disabilities*. Baltimore, MD: Brookes; 1989.

Anderson SW, Demasio AR, Demasio H. Troubled letters but not numbers. Domain specific cognitive impairments following damage in frontal cortex. *Brain*. 1990;113:749–766.

Baillieux H, Vandervliet EJ, Manto M, Parizel PM, Deyn PP, Marien P. Developmental dyslexia and widespread activation across the cerebellar hemispheres. *Brain Lang*. Nov 3, 2008; [E-pub].

Boder E. Developmental dyslexia: A diagnostic approach used on three atypical reading-spelling patterns. *Dev Med Child Neurol*. 1973;15:663–687.

Cohen M, et al. Neuropathological abnormalities in developmental dysphasia. *Ann Neurol*. 1989;25:567–570.

Del'Homme M, Kim TS, Loo SK, Yang MH, Smalley SL. Familial association and frequency of learning disabilities in ADHD sibling pair families. *J Abnorm Child Psychol*. 2007;35:55–62.

Denckla MB. Introduction to learning disorders. In: Millichap JG, ed. *Progress in Pediatric Neurology II*. Chicago, IL: PNB Publishers; 1994.

Ecalle J, Magnan A, Bouchafa H, Gombert JE. Computer-based training with ortho-phonological units in dyslexic children: new investigations. *Dyslexia*. July 21, 2008;[E-pub].

Fernald GM. *Remedial Techniques in Basic School Subjects*. New York: McGraw-Hill; 1947.

Fischel JE, Whitehurst GJ, Caulfield MB, DeBaryshe B. Language growth in children with expressive language delay. *Pediatrics*. 1989;83:218–227.

Flynn JM, Deering WM. Subtypes of dyslexia: Investigation of Boder's system using quantitative neurophysiology. *Dev Med Child Neurol*. 1989;31:215–223.

Frolich J, Dopfner M. The treatment of attention-deficit/hyperactivity disorders with polyunsaturated fatty acids – an effective treatment alternative? *Z Kinder Jugendpsychiatr Psychother*. 2008;36:109–116.

Galaburda AM, et al. Developmental dyslexia: four consecutive patients with cortical anomalies. *Ann Neurol*. 1985;18:222.

Geiger G, Lettvin JY. Peripheral and central vision of dyslexic adults. *N Engl J Med*. 1987;316:1238.

Gillingham A, Stillman B. *Remedial Training for Children with Specific Language Disability in Reading, Spelling and Penmanship*. Cambridge, MA: The Educator's Publishing Service; 1956.

Given BK, Wasserman JD, Chari SA, Beattie K, Eden GF. A randomized, controlled study of computer-based intervention in middle school struggling readers. *Brain Lang*. 2008;106:83–97.

Hartlage LC. Neuropsychological assessment techniques. In: Reynolds CR, Gutkin TB (eds). *The Handbook of School Psychology*. New York: Wiley; 1981.

Heilman KM, et al. Developmental dyslexia: a motor-articulatory feedback hypothesis. *Ann Neurol*. 1996;39:407–412.

Hoeft F, Hernandez A, McMillon G, et al. Neural basis of dyslexia: a comparison between dyslexic and nondyslexic children equated for reading ability. *J Neurosci*. 2006;26:10700–10708.

Humphreys P, et al. Developmental dyslexia in women: neuropathological findings in three patients. *Ann Neurol*. 1990;28:727–738.

Hynd GW, et al. Dyslexia and corpus callosum morphology. *Arch Neurol*. 1995;52:32–38.

Hynd G, Cohen M. *Dyslexia. Neuropsychological Theory, Research, and Clinical Differentiations*. New York: Grune & Stratton; 1983.

Kairaluoma L, Narhi V, Ahonen T, Westerholm J, Aro M. Do fatty acids help in overcoming reading difficulties? A double-blind, placebo-controlled study of the effects of eicosapentaenoic acid and carnosine supplementation on children with dyslexia. *Child Care Health Dev*. Oct 22, 2008;[E-pub].

Klassen AF, Miller A, Fine S. Health-related quality of life in children and adolescents who have a diagnosis of attention-deficit/hyperactivity disorder. *Pediatrics*. 2004;114:e541–e547.

Lajiness-O'Neill R, Akamine Y, Bowyer SM. Treatment effects of fast ForWord demonstrated by magnetoencephalography (MEG) in a child with developmental dyslexia. *Neurocase*. 2007;13:390–401.

Lehmkuhle S, et al. A defective visual pathway in children with reading disability. *N Engl J Med*. 1993;328:989–996.

Levy F, et al. Twin-sibling differences in ADHD children with reading and speech problems. *J Child Psychol Psychiatry*. 1996;37:569–578.

Loonen MCB, van Dongen HR. Acquired childhood aphasia. Outcome 1 year after onset. *Arch Neurol*. 1990;47:1324–1328.

Magnan A, Ecalle J, Veuillet E, Collet L. The effects of an audio-visual training program in dyslexic children. *Dyslexia*. 2004;10:131–140.

Magnan A, et al. *Dyslexia*. 2004;10:1–10.

Mayes SD, Calhoun SL, Crowell EW. Learning disabilities and ADHD: overlapping spectrum disorders. *J Learn Disabil*. 2000;33:417–424.

Merzenich MM, et al. Temporal processing deficits of language-learning impaired children ameliorated by training. *Science*. 1996;271:77–81.

Millichap NM. Dyslexia: Theories of Causation and Methods of Management. A Historical Perspective. Loyola University of Chicago, Masters Degree Thesis, 1986.

Millichap JG ed. *Progress in Pediatric Neurology III*. Chicago, IL: PNB Publishers; 1997.

Millichap NM, Millichap JG. *Dyslexia: As the Educator and Neurologist Read It*. Springfield, IL: Charles C Thomas; 1986.

Nielsen JM. *Agnosia, Apraxia, Aphasia. Their Value in Cerebral Localization*. New York: Hafner Publ Comp, Paul B Hoeber; 1965.

Orton ST. *Reading, Writing, and Speech Problems in Children: A Presentation of Certain Types of Disorders in the Development of the Language Faculty*. New York: Norton; 1937.

Pastor PN, Reuben CA. Diagnosed attention deficit hyperactivity disorder and learning disability: United States, 2004–2006. *Vital Health Stat 10*. 2008 Jul;237:1–14.

Paulesu E, et al. A disconnection syndrome hypothesis for developmental dyslexia. *Brain*. 1996;119:143–157.

Price CJ, et al. Brain activity during reading. The effects of exposure duration and task. *Brain*. 1994;117:1255–1269.

Richardson AJ. Omega-3 fatty acids in ADHD and related neurodevelopmental disorders. *Int Rev Psychiatry*. 2006;18:155–172.

Richardson AJ, Montgomery P. The Oxford-Durham study: a randomized, controlled trial of supplementation with fatty acids in children with developmental coordination disorder. *Pediatrics*. 2005;115:1360–1366.

Salmelin R, et al. Impaired visual word processing in dyslexia revealed with magnetoencephalography. *Ann Neurol*. 1996;40:157–162.

Schultz RT, et al. Brain morphology in normal and dyslexic children: The influence of sex and age. *Ann Neurol*. 1994;35:732–742.

Schumacher J, Konig IR, Schroder T, et al. Further evidence for a susceptibility locus contributing to reading disability on chromosome 15q15-q21. *J Psychiatr Genet*. 2008;8:137–142.

Seidman LJ, et al. A pilot study of neuropsychological function in girls with ADHD. *J Am Acad Child Adolesc Psychiatry*. 1997;36:366–373.

Shalev RS, Gross-Tsur V. Developmental dyscalculia and medical assessment. *J Learn Disabil*. 1993;26:134–137.

Shaywitz BA, Fletcher JM, Shaywitz SE. Defining and classifying learning disabilities and attention-deficit/hyperactivity disorder. *J Child Neurol*. 1995;10(Suppl 1):S50–S57.

Shaywitz SE, Shaywitz BA. Paying attention to reading: the neurobiology of reading and dyslexia. *Dev Psychopathol*. 2008;20:1329–1349.

Stevenson J, et al. A twin study of genetic influences on reading and spelling ability and disability. *J Child Psychol Psychiatry*. 1987;28:229–247.

Stevenson J, Langley K, Pay H, et al. Attention deficit hyperactivity disorder with reading disabilities: preliminary genetic findings on the involvement of the ADRAZA gene. *J Child Psychol Psychiatry*. 2005;46:1081–1088.

Strauss EW, Lehtinen L. *Psychopathology and Education of the Brain-Injured Child*. New York: Grune and Stratton; 1947.

Tallal P, et al. Language comprehension in language-learning impaired children improved with acoustically modified speech. *Science*. 1996;271:81–84.

Ta'ir J, et al. Profound developmental dyscalculia: evidence for a cardinal/ordinal skills acquisition device. *Brain Cogn*. 1997;35:184–206.

Tonnessen FE, et al. Dyslexia, left-handedness, and immune disorders. *Arch Neurol*. 1993;50: 411–416.

Veuillet E, Magnan A, Ecalle J, Thai-Van H, Collet L. Auditory processing disorder in children with reading disabilities: effect of audiovisual training. *Brain*. 2007;130:2915–2928.

World Federation of Neurology Definition. In Waites L. Definition of dyslexia. *Can Med Assoc J*. 1968;99:37.

Chapter 7
Tics, Tourette Syndrome, Seizures, and Headaches

Neurological disorders that sometimes complicate the syndrome of attention deficit hyperactivity disorder include tics and Tourette syndrome, seizures and headaches. Causes underlying the ADHD may also be responsible for these disorders or, alternatively, drugs used in the treatment of ADHD may result in neurological side-effects. Special tests, including an EEG and CT or MRI, may be necessary to uncover the cause and determine the appropriate therapy. The recognition and diagnosis of associated neurological disorders is important for the optimal management of ADHD.

Tics and Tourette Syndome

Tic or habit spasm is an involuntary, recurrent twitch or motor movement (motor tic) or a grunt or vocalization (vocal tic). *Simple motor tics* involve the eyes, as in eye blinking (blepharospasm), the face (grimacing) and the head, neck, and shoulders (jerking, twisting, and shrugging movements). *Simple vocal tics* include throat-clearing, grunting, sniffing, and barking. *Complex motor tics* are gestures, jumping, and touching objects. *Complex vocal tics* are utterances of obscene language (copro-lalia), repeating words or phrases, sometimes out of context (palilalia), and repeating words said by another person (echolalia). Sometimes precipitated by a physical or emotional stimulus, the tic can be controlled partially by will and is infrequent during sleep. It is exaggerated by stress and fatigue and lessened by diverting the child's attention.

Tics can be *transient* or *chronic,* and *definite* (observed by the physician) or only by *history or report* (not observed by the physician). *Transient tic disorder* lasts for at least two weeks, but no longer than one year. *Chronic tic disorder* is manifested by either motor or vocal tics, occurring intermittently for more than one year.

Tourette syndrome, named after a French neurologist, Georges Gilles de la Tourette, is characterized by chronic tics, both motor and vocal, persisting for longer than one year. Tourette first described his syndrome in 1885, with a preliminary report in 1884. An English-language translation of the report is provided by Lajonchere et al. (1996).

J.G. Millichap, *Attention Deficit Hyperactivity Disorder Handbook*,
DOI 10.1007/978-1-4419-1397-5_7, © Springer Science+Business Media, LLC 2010

Prevalence of Tourette Syndrome

The incidence of reported cases of Tourette syndrome (TS) before the 1960s was low, and the disorder was generally omitted from the index of textbooks of neurology. Increased public awareness of TS and the recognition of organic in addition to functional psychiatric causes have led to an increase in apparent prevalence. The frequency of transient tics in childhood is variably quoted at 4–16%. A study involving school children from *Monroe County, NY*, conducted at the *University of Rochester Medical Center, NY*, detected 41 with Tourette syndrome (TS), with an estimated prevalence of 29 per 100,000 (Caine et al., 1988).

In the Monroe County study, TS was a mild disorder in more than one half the cases, and medication was required in less than half. Thirty-seven were boys and four were girls. Eleven (27%) had ADHD, and methylphenidate appeared to be the cause in 10 (25%). In addition to simple motor and vocal tics, 20 (50%) children had complex vocalizations including coprolalia, echolalia, and stuttering. Twenty (50%) also had obsessive-compulsive symptoms, including touching or repetitive placing of objects.

The remarkably large percentage of patients with TS related to ADHD and treatment with methylphenidate (25% in this series) might explain the increased awareness of Tourette syndrome since the 1960s, when the use of Ritalin® became widespread. A questionnaire mailed to pediatric neurologists to determine their usage of methylphenidate in the treatment of ADHD revealed that 5% of children who were treated with methylphenidate developed tics (Millichap, 1997).

Causes of Tics and Tourette Syndrome

Originally considered an emotional, compulsive, or psychiatric disorder, recent research emphasizes an organic, neurologic basis for tic disorders. Both genetic and acquired factors are invoked. Acquired causes include encephalitis, head trauma, neonatal asphyxia, and an abnormal reaction to streptococcal infection. Congenital anomalies of brain development have been demonstrated in some cases, and tics in adults can occur rarely as manifestations of cerebral tumors, multiple sclerosis, Huntington's, Alzheimer's, and Creutzfeldt-Jakob diseases.

In children with ADHD, tics may be precipitated by stimulant medications such as methylphenidate (Ritalin®) or amphetamines (Dexedrine,® Adderall®). Dietary stimulants including coffee, tea, and chocolate may also exacerbate tics. A neurochemical mechanism for the stimulant-induced tic seems likely. Methylphenidate is probably the most common precipitating cause of tics and Tourette syndrome among school-age children.

Other factors found to influence the frequency and severity of tics include hormonal changes, thermal stress, voluntary and purposeful compulsions, and stimulus-induced behaviors or "impulsions." Menstrual cycle fluctuations in the frequency of tics were noted in adolescent girls with Tourette syndrome followed at the *Children's Hospital of Wisconsin, Milwaukee, WI* (Schwabe and Konkol, 1992). Tics increased with menarche, the beginning of menstruation and before each menstrual period; they decreased after menstruation.

A 17 year-old boy with Tourette syndrome had more frequent tics during warmer weather, during fever, or after vigorous exercise (Lombroso et al., 1991). In a study of patients' perceptions of tics, two thirds of a group of 60 patients diagnosed with Tourette syndrome thought their movements and vocalizations were intentional and under voluntary control. This perception of the nature of tics is contrary to the prevailing neurological theory of an involuntary movement disorder, only partially controlled by will (Lang, 1991). The term "impulsions" is used to describe tics and obsessive-compulsive behaviorisms induced by stimuli such as tightness in the chest or tingling sensations (sensory tic) or in response to another person coughing (reflex tic) (Eapen et al., 1994).

Genetics of Tourette Syndrome and Tic Disorders

An autosomal dominant mode of transmission from both maternal and paternal sides of the family is suggested by genetic studies, but the identification of a responsible gene remains elusive. Maternally transmitted cases have an earlier age of onset (Eapen et al., 1997). Studies in monozygotic twins with tic disorders have shown a concordance rate of less than 100% and a variability of tic severity among family members, ranging from simple transient tic disorder to severe and persistent Tourette syndrome (TS). The TS gene is variably expressed as TS, transient tic disorder, or chronic tic disorder (Kurlan et al., 1988).

Children with a first-degree relative with Tourette syndrome have an increased risk of developing tic disorders, and they are also more likely to have obsessive-compulsive and attention deficit disorders (Carter et al., 1994). Environmental factors in addition to inheritance play a role in the causation of tics and TS, and the neurotransmitter dopamine is involved in the mechanism of these disorders.

Structural Brain Abnormalities and Tourette Syndrome

Reduction in volume and asymmetries in size of the basal ganglia, and increases in the size of certain regions of the corpus callosum are defined by analysis of MRIs of children and adolescents with Tourette syndrome (TS). Using special imaging techniques, Singer HS, Denckla MB, and colleagues at *Johns Hopkins University* found, in contrast to those with TS alone, children with TS and ADHD show decreases in size of the corpus callosum and changes involving the basal ganglia (1993, 1996). Tourette syndrome and ADHD may result from distinct neurodevelopmental processes, representing different degrees of expression of the same gene.

Acute basal ganglia enlargement was correlated with severity of obsessive-compulsive disorder (OCD) and tics following a hemolytic streptococcal throat infection in a 12-year-old boy. Serum antibodies against the basal ganglia and anti-streptolysin titers were elevated in children with ADHD complicated by tics or other movement disorders (Kiessling et al., 1993). Antibiotic and blood plasmapheresis treatments resulted in a rapid shrinkage of the basal ganglia and improvement in the OCD and tics (Giedd et al., 1996). The swelling of the basal ganglia might be explained by an inflammation and edema, secondary to a reaction between antibodies and invading bacteria. Tics and OCD represent in some cases an autoimmune reaction to streptococcal infection, and immunological and antibiotic therapies may be beneficial.

Neuroanatomical studies using MRI measurements show correlations between volume changes in the basal ganglia and corpus callosum and the severity of Tourette syndrome. These anatomical changes can be developmental and genetic and, in some cases, result from infection and an autoimmune reaction. Other environmental factors altering the function of the basal ganglia and resulting in tics include head trauma and encephalitis (Millichap, 1994).

Relation of Streptococcal Infection to Tics and OCD

The association between Group A b-hemolytic streptococcal infection (GABHS) and the development of tics and Tourette syndrome (TS) is considered a pediatric autoimmune disorder, similar to Sydenham's chorea and rheumatic fever. The mechanism of chorea and streptococcal-induced TS involves GABHS antibodies that cross-react with the basal ganglia and result in the characteristic movement disorders and antineuronal antibody formation. Tics and TS as a sequel to Sydenham's chorea are not a novel finding. The association was recognized more than 60 years ago by Guttmann (1927) and reviewed by Wilson (1955).

Tics with an autoimmune mechanism are often associated with obsessive-compulsive disorder. Evidence of a recent streptococcal infection and persistent elevation of antistreptolysin O titers may indicate the need for prophylactic penicillin. The use of antibiotics to prevent future exacerbations of tics is controversial and requires further study.

Evidence for Encephalitis as a Cause of Tourette Syndrome

A six-year-old girl who developed a Tourette-like syndrome following herpes encephalitis was treated at *Walter Reed Army Medical Center, Washington, DC, and Johns Hopkins University, Baltimore, MD* (Northram and Singer, 1991). At two weeks after recovery from the encephalitis and discharge from hospital she developed eye blinking and sudden, rapidly recurrent, purposeless movements and vocalizations. The motor tics were characterized by facial grimacing, head twitching, and shoulder shrugging plus eye rolling, facial contortions, jumping, touching objects and body parts, and obscene gestures. Vocal tics included grunting, sniffing, and snorting sounds. Recovery followed several weeks of therapy with pimozide (Orap®). MRIs showed a hemorrhage in the basal ganglia and temporal lobe of the brain. An EEG showed slow waves over the same temporal lobe region, indicating destruction or swelling of brain tissue.

Older textbooks of neurology refer to tics and Tourette-like syndrome as complications of encephalitis lethargica and, like the hyperactive behavior syndrome (ADHD), these movement disorders were a delayed result of the influenza epidemic of 1918. Opinions favored an organic, brain-damage cause for the encephalitis-induced tic, while other tic disorders unassociated with encephalitis were regarded as compulsive habit spasms and symptoms of psychogenic illness (Wilson, 1955). The more recent medical literature invokes encephalitis as just one of a number of acquired causes for Tourette syndrome.

Tourette Syndrome and Risk of Learning Disabilities

In a study of 138 children with Tourette's syndrome (TS) at the *University of Rochester, NY*, a diagnosis of specific learning disorder was made in 30 (22%). Of the remaining 108, 36 (33%) had significant school problems, including grade retention and special education placement. The association of ADHD with TS was a significant predictor of academic problems (Abwender et al., 1996).

More than 50% of children with Tourette syndrome are affected by specific learning disabilities or other academic problems. Tics themselves are not the reason for the school problems, but rather the associated "comorbid" ADHD. These findings confirm those of the Johns Hopkins investigators, who report that children with TS complicated by ADHD have a 32% risk of developing a specific learning disability whereas those with TS alone have no academic problems (Schuerholz et al., 1996).

Children with either TS or chronic tic disorder suffered from learning disabilities and lowered academic achievement, in a study at the *Massachusetts General Hospital, Boston* (Spencer et al., 1995). Children with TS differed from control subjects in having increased rates of comorbid ADHD, obsessive-compulsive disorder (OCD), mood disorders (depression, bipolar disorder), antisocial disorders (conduct and oppositional defiant disorder (ODD)), and anxiety disorders. TS patients differed from tic disorder patients in having higher rates of OCD and ODD. TS and chronic tic disorder are related diseases, TS being more severe than chronic tic disorder. Comorbidity with ADHD, occurring in 50% of TS patients, causes more disability than the motor tics alone.

Bipolar Disorder and Tourette Syndrome

The incidence of bipolar disorder (manic or depressive symptoms) among children and adolescents with Tourette syndrome is four times higher than that expected by chance. Boys are at greater risk than girls, in a ratio of 5:1. The frequency and intensity of motor and vocal tics increase with manic symptoms and decrease with depressive symptoms. These findings were reported by the *North Dakota Longitudinal Tourette Syndrome Surveillance Project,* in which 205 patients were followed and 15 developed comorbid bipolar disorder, some with histories of ADHD (Kerbeshian et al., 1995).

Common neurochemical mechanisms, involving noradrenergic, dopaminergic, and serotonergic pathways in the basal ganglia, and genetic factors are invoked as explanations for the comorbidity of TS, bipolar disorder, and ADHD.

Treatment of Tourette Syndrome Complicating ADHD

If tics or Tourette syndrome occur in association with ADHD or are known to affect other members of the immediate family, stimulant medications and caffeine-containing drinks should generally be avoided. An exception may be the child who is benefiting from immediate-release methylphenidate (MPH-IR) and the ADHD is complicated by a chronic tic disorder.

In a study of 71 children (ages 6–12 years) with ADHD and Tourette syndrome or chronic motor tic disorder treated with MPH (0.1, 0.3, and 0.5 mg/kg) and placebo twice daily for 2 weeks each, double-blind, MPH-IR effectively suppressed ADHD, ODD, and peer aggression disorders, without altering the overall severity of tic disorder. Teacher ratings showed a decrease in frequency and severity of the tic disorder, whereas the physician ratings revealed an increase in simple but not in complex motor movements, with MPH doses of 0.3 and 0.5 mg/kg. The researchers concluded that MPH-IR is not contraindicated as short-term therapy for children with ADHD and chronic tic disorder, but treatment should be carefully monitored to exclude possible tic exacerbations in susceptible individuals (Gadow et al., 2007).

Larger doses of MPH resulted in minimal increased effectiveness but a greater likelihood of tic exacerbation and adverse effects on heart rate, blood pressure, and weight gain. An improved tic control reported by teachers in the classroom may be explained by a student's ability to suppress tics in the stigmatizing school environment. Evaluations in multiple environments are necessary to determine the true frequency and severity of a tic disorder. Children with ADHD who develop tics during treatment with methylphenidate or other stimulant should receive an alternative type of medication, an antihypertensive drug, clonidine, or guanfacine. The suitability of the non-stimulant atomoxetine in patients with tics is under investigation.

Atomoxetine HCl (Strattera®), a nonstimulant, is a selective norepinephrine reuptake inhibitor for the treatment of ADHD. Atomoxetine is widely used as an alternative to stimulants in children with ADHD complicated by tics or TS. In addition to children with ADHD and tics, atomoxetine is preferred to the stimulant class of compounds in children with ADHD complicated by a tendency to seizures, an abnormal EEG, or sleep disorder. Contraindications include recent treatment with monoamine oxidase inhibitors (MAOI), history of depression or suicidal thoughts, narrow angle glaucoma, or allergic reaction to atomoxetine. Parents are warned of a possible risk of suicidal thinking and the need to discontinue treatment. Elevation of liver enzymes is reported rarely. Tachycardia and elevation of blood pressure may occur but less frequently than with stimulants. An electrocardiogram and cardiac consultation are advisable, if a heart murmur is detected or serious heart disease is reported in family members.

Recent isolated reports of tic exacerbation and precipitation during atomoxetine treatment of ADHD introduce a note of caution and need for frequent monitoring. In two case reports, tics that developed after the introduction or following an increase in dose of atomoxetine did not resolve when treatment was discontinued. Alternative interventional therapy such as clonidine was finally successful in the control of tics (Parraga et al., 2007; Sears and Patel, 2008).

Clonidine (Catapres®) is an a_2-adrenergic agonist. It lowers blood pressure by activating receptors in the brain stem, suppressing the outflow of sympathetic nervous system activity. The release of norepinephrine from peripheral nerve endings and the plasma concentration of norepinephrine are also decreased, effects that might explain the benefits observed in children with ADHD and tics.

In children of 5 years of age and older with ADHD and tics, the usual starting dose is one half of a 0.1 mg tablet given by mouth at night, 1 h before bedtime. Drowsiness is the most common side effect, and the dose may have to be modified to one-quarter tablet nightly if drowsiness persists during the school day. Dryness of the mouth is a side effect that occurs in 30–40% of adults while taking clonidine but is rarely mentioned by children treated with the drug.

Unlike methylphenidate, the response to clonidine is slow, often delayed for up to two weeks, and doses are given daily on school days and at weekends. Parents are advised to be patient, and teachers should not expect dramatic improvements in attention, focus, or behavior when the drug is first introduced. After two weeks, one-quarter tablet after breakfast is added daily if symptoms of ADHD and tics persist. Further increments in dosage are made slowly, usually at 7-day intervals and generally to a maximum of 0.15 mg daily, given in divided amounts 2 or 3 times a day, depending on the individual response and reports of drowsiness. The pulse and blood pressure should be monitored regularly, and withdrawals of this drug should be slow, to prevent rebound in blood pressure. An electrocardiogram should be obtained before starting treatment, if cardiac problems are suspected. To avoid cardiac and blood pressure adverse effects, combination treatment of clonidine with a stimulant or tricyclic antidepressant is not recommended.

A transdermal product is available, Catapres-TTS-1®, applied to the skin of the upper arm, once every 7 days. I have no experience with the patch and cannot recommend its use. About 15–20% of adult patients develop a skin rash or contact dermatitis when using the clonidine transdermal patch (Goodman & Gilman, 1996). If used in children with ADHD, the patch should be tightly controlled and the blood pressure and pulse closely monitored.

Guanfacine (Tenex®) is an alternative antihypertensive agent to clonidine. Guanfacine is a more selective a2-adrenoceptor agonist than clonidine, binding preferentially to receptors in the prefrontal cortex. It has a longer plasma half-life and is less sedating and less hypotensive. The initial dosage in children of school age is one quarter to one half the 1.0 mg tablet daily, given 1 h before bedtime. Drowsiness is the most common side effect, and increments in dosage of one-quarter tablet are made slowly, at 7–14 day intervals, usually to a maximum of 1.5 mg daily in 2 or 3 divided amounts. The same precautions are observed with guanfacine as with clonidine.

In one study of guanfacine (1.5 mg daily) in 10 children with TS and ADHD, treated at *Yale and Johns Hopkins Universities,* significant improvements in attention were observed in continuous performance tasks, and the severity of motor and phonic tics was also decreased. Side effects included transient fatigue, headaches, and drowsiness (Chappell et al., 1995).

Guanfacine XR. A multicenter, double-blind, placebo-controlled trial of an extended release formulation of guanfacine in ADHD included 345 patients aged 6–17 years randomly assigned to 1 of 3 guanfacine dosage groups (2, 3, or 4 mg/each AM) or placebo for 8 weeks. All groups of children taking guanfacine showed significant improvement in hyperactivity/impulsivity and inattentiveness subscales of the ADHD Rating Scale IV, Clinical Global Impression, Parent's Global Assessment, and Conners' Parent and Teacher Rating Scales-Revised. Adverse events included headache, somnolence, fatigue, abdominal pain, and sedation. Treatment was discontinued because of somnolence in 4.2%, sedation in 3.5%, and headache in 1.5%. Blood pressure and pulse rate decreased as dosages were increased, by a maximum of –10.1 mm Hg and –8 bpm, respectively. Seven patients discontinued treatment because of ECG abnormalities, 4 with QTc interval prolongation, one in each treatment and dosage group. Mean changes in height and weight were unremarkable. Guanfacine XR was considered safe and effective in treatment of ADHD (Biederman et al., 2008).

Guanfacine XR may prove superior to the immediate release preparation and is effective in a once daily dosage. Provided sedation is not a problem, guanfacine may be preferred to stimulant medication in the younger child with hyperactive behavior and ODD. Pretreatment cardiac evaluation with ECG and regular heart monitoring are advisable.

Other medications sometimes advised in treatment of Tourette syndrome include risperidone and clomipramine. Side effects must be monitored carefully. Children with transient tics rarely need medication. Parents are advised to withdraw caffeine-containing drinks and chocolate. The attention of the child should be diverted away from the recognition of the tics if possible, and anxiety-provoking situations at school and at home should be avoided.

Seizures and ADHD

Epilepsies Comorbid with ADHD in Children

Seizures of the absence or complex partial types may be the cause of "daydreaming" or episodes of confusion and inattention noted by the teacher, psychologist, or parent of a child with ADHD.

Indications for an electroencephalogram in ADHD children include one or more of the following risk factors for epilepsy:

• History of convulsion in early childhood;
• History of epilepsy in a sibling or parent;

- History of head trauma, encephalitis, or meningitis; or
- Episodes of staring, confusion, fear, uncontrolled rage, or laughter.

Absence seizures are accompanied by a generalized EEG discharge whereas partial seizures originate with a focal, localized epileptiform discharge. An abnormal, epileptiform EEG associated with episodic symptoms may be diagnostic of seizures. In children with comorbid epilepsy/ADHD, a trial of antiepileptic medication may be indicated before stimulants are prescribed for ADHD.

Prevalence and Significance of EEG Abnormalities with ADHD

Electroencephalographic abnormalities in 7 studies of non-epileptic children with ADHD are reviewed and results are summarized in Table 7.1. Overall, the incidence of epileptiform discharges is 23.1%. Two studies that included prolonged video-polysomnographic recordings found EEG seizure discharges of 40 and 53% patients. When patients with polysomnograms are excluded and routine EEG results of 5 studies are tabulated, the mean incidence of epileptiform EEGs in children with ADHD is 13.7%. Prolonged sleep recordings are probably more indicative of the true incidence of epileptiform EEG. Summaries of results of the 7 studies are as follows:

Table 7.1 Electroencephalographic abnormalities in non-epileptic children with ADHD

References	Patients (no.)	Epileptiform EEGs (%)
Millichap (1977)	100	7
Hughes et al. (2000)	176	30.1
Hemmer et al. (2001)	234	15.4
Richer et al. (2002)	347	6.1
Castaneda-Cabrero et al. (2003)	15	40[a]
Silvestri et al. (2007)	42	53[a]
Fonseca et al. (2008)	30	10
Total EEGs	944	23.1%

[a]Polysomnographic studies

EEGs in 100 children with ADHD studied consecutively showed abnormal discharges compatible with epilepsy in 7%. Another 19% patients had moderate irregularities indicative of brain dysfunction, not specific for epilepsy (Millichap, 1977). An abnormal EEG is not always an indication for antiepileptic (AED) therapy, but when associated with episodic symptoms suggestive of seizures, a trial of AED treatment may be warranted.

In a study of 176 children with ADHD, EEG recordings showed epileptiform activity in 30.1%. Seizure discharges were mainly focal (usually occipital or temporal), and generalized bilaterally synchronous spike and wave complexes occurred in 11 (6.25%) children. The EEGs were completely normal in 27.8% (Hughes et al., 2000).

In a study to determine the risks of stimulant therapy in non-epileptic children with ADHD, EEGs performed in 234 patients found 15.4% with epileptiform abnormalities and 84.6% with normal or non-epileptiform records. Of 36 patients with abnormal EEGs, 40% had rolandic spikes and 60% had focal abnormalities. Of 205 patients treated with stimulant therapy for ADHD, seizures occurred in 1 of 175 patients with a normal EEG (incidence 0.6%) and in 3 of 30 with epileptiform EEGs (incidence 10%). Seizures occurred in 2 of 12 (16.7%) children with rolandic spikes. An epileptiform EEG in neurologically normal children with ADHD is predictive of a significantly increased risk of seizures associated with stimulant therapy (Hemmer et al., 2001).

An EEG performed in 347 children 5–16 years of age referred with ADHD showed epileptiform discharges in 6.1% ± 1.3%. This was significantly higher than an epileptiform EEG prevalence rate of 3.5 ± 0.6% observed in a study of 3,726 normal school-aged children ($P < 0.025$) (Richer et al., 2002). The epileptiform abnormality was present only with activation procedures in 6 patients (2 with hyperventilation and 4 photic stimulation). Only 3 of the 21 ADHD children with epileptiform abnormalities developed a seizure disorder. The authors concluded that the clinical utility of routine EEG in the diagnosis of a comorbid seizure disorder in children with ADHD is limited.

Of 15 children referred with ADHD, the waking EEG showed epileptiform discharges in 2 patients (spike and wave paroxysms in the left temporoparietal region and spike wave discharges during hyperventilation). A polysomnographic study revealed seizure discharges in 4 patients (1 with continuous spike wave trace during slow sleep (CSWS), 2 showing paroxysmal spike and slow waves in the temporoparietal region with secondary generalization, and 1 case with frequent generalized paroxysmal slow waves in all phases of sleep). A polysomnographic study is recommended in certain cases of ADHD (Castaneda-Cabrero et al., 2003).

In 42 ADHD outpatients (35 boys and 7 girls) referred to a sleep clinic for all night video-polysomnography, 86% had sleep disorders, and of these 26% were restless leg syndrome. Interictal epileptiform discharges (IEDs) were recorded in 53% of ADHD children; 28% were centro-temporal spikes, 12.5% frontal spikes, 9.3% temporo-occipital spikes, and 2.3% generalized spike-wave. Nocturnal seizures occurred in 3 patients, 2 with rolandic spikes, and 1 with left frontal slowing on the EEG. The presence of seizures or IEDs is correlated with cognitive and visual-spatial memory deficits, while sleep disorders have a stronger adverse effect on behavioral problems with ADHD (Silvestri et al., 2007).

Epileptiform EEG activity was found in 3 (10%) of 30 children with ADHD. Compared to 30 sex- and age-matched healthy controls, the ADHD group showed significantly greater absolute delta and theta activity on quantitative EEG (Fonseca et al., 2008) (Fig. 7.1).

The EEG is helpful in the differentiation of epilepsy and daydreaming of the inattentive child with ADHD. The test is useful not only in diagnosis but also in treatment of learning and behavior disorders. Central nervous system stimulants and some antidepressants may precipitate seizures and should be used with caution in children with seizure activity in the EEG.

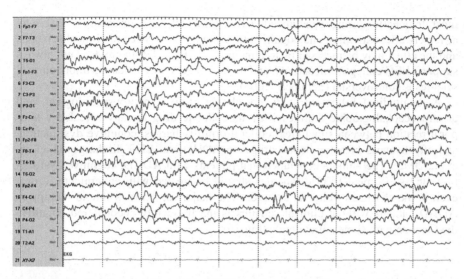

Fig. 7.1 EEG of an 8-year-old boy with ADHD showing frequent focal epileptiform discharges from either central area, maximal left, without concurrent clinical seizures. The record is compatible with that of benign focal, rolandic epilepsy. (*Courtesy of Cynthia Stack MD, Director of Neurophysiology Laboratory, Children's Memorial Hospital, Chicago*)

Stimulant Therapy in Comorbid Epilepsy/ADHD

In a study designed to determine the safety and effectiveness of methylphenidate (MPH) in 25 children with comorbid epilepsy and ADHD, all receiving antiepileptic drugs (AEDs), 5 continued to have seizures after MPH was introduced, 3 with an increase in attacks and 2 with no change or less. Of 20 patients whose seizures were controlled by AEDs, none had attacks while taking MPH (Gross-Tsur et al., 1997). The authors conclude that MPH is safe in children with comorbid epilepsy/ADHD whose seizures are controlled with AEDs. MPH should be used with caution in patients whose seizures are AED refractory.

A more recent review concludes that the addition of MPH is safe in children with ADHD and epilepsy whose seizures are controlled with AEDs (Tan and Appleton, 2005). In contrast, children with ADHD and subclinical epileptiform EEGs may develop seizures with the introduction of MPH (Hemmer et al., 2001). The incidence of seizures following MPH was 16.7% in children with ADHD complicated by EEG centro-temporal (rolandic) spikes compared to 0.6% in a group of ADHD patients with normal EEGs.

Epileptiform EEG and Transient Cognitive Deficit

Brief cognitive deficits (*transient cognitive impairment [TCI]*) are reported in patients with ADHD complicated by subclinical epileptiform EEG abnormalities, most frequently during generalized 3-Hz spike-and-wave discharges. TCI may adversely affect attention and cognitive function in the absence of clinical seizures, and the effect may be reversed by treatment with AEDs. Treatment does not always suppress EEG epileptiform activity, and the use of AEDs in patients without clinical seizures is controversial (Schubert, 2005).

A longitudinal follow-up study correlating clinical, neuropsychological, and electroencephalographic features with antiepileptic drug therapy revealed a temporal relation between subclinical epileptiform discharges, cognitive dysfunction, and effectiveness of antiepileptic drugs on ADHD and EEG discharges (Laporte et al., 2002). The authors concluded that patients with ADHD, cognitive dysfunction, and subclinical EEG discharges should be treated with antiepileptic drugs, even in the absence of clinical seizures. The major reason to withhold therapy in ADHD patients without clinical seizures is the frequently encountered cognitive dysfunction with some antiepileptic drugs.

Cognitive Effects of Antiepileptic Drugs

AEDs have variable effects on attention, learning, and behavior. Phenobarbital, gabapentin, and topiramate are associated with cognitive impairments, whereas carbamazepine and lamotrigine may improve attention and behavior. Phenytoin and oxcarbazepine have no documented effects on symptoms of ADHD. Very few controlled studies of the cognitive side effects of antiepileptic drugs are reported, but improvement in cognition and behavior often follows the withdrawal of medication (Nordli, 2004; Loring and Meador, 2004; Hessen et al., 2006).

EEG Localization, Epilepsy, and Learning Disability

The localization of the EEG abnormal discharge is helpful in the differentiation of learning disorders associated with ADHD. Attentional difficulties in children with some types of epilepsy are related to dysfunction in the right cerebral hemisphere and are associated with impaired visuo-spatial processing. Left hemisphere dysfunction causes language-related learning disabilities. The side of the epileptic EEG focus is linked to the type of learning deficit (Piccirilli et al., 1994).

Prevalence of ADHD in Children with Epilepsy

One in 5 children with epilepsy may have ADHD, according to one report (Gross-Tsur et al., 1997). A recent study involving 203 patients found approximately 60% of children with epilepsy have either ADHD-Inattentive subtype (ADHD-I) or ADHD-Combined Inattentive, Hyperactive-Impulsive subtype (ADHD-C)

(Sherman et al., 2007). Inattention was diagnosed in 40% and hyperactivity-impulsivity in 18% of children with severe epilepsy. Epilepsy patients were pre- or post-surgical candidates; 74% localization related and 17% generalized epilepsies. ADHD-I was associated with a greater frequency of localization-related epilepsy and more frequent use of antiepileptic drugs with cognitive side effects (benzo-diazepines, topiramate, phenobarbital). Quality of life was impaired twofold in children with severe epilepsy complicated by ADHD-I, and fourfold with ADHD-C comorbidity, when compared to non-ADHD/epilepsy patients.

A review of ADHD and epilepsy that includes 108 references concludes that findings are difficult to interpret because of lack of conformity in ages of patients, severity and types of epilepsy, differences in behavior rating scales, and effects of antiepileptic drugs (Schubert, 2005). Most studies reported that impairment of attention was more likely with generalized epilepsies than with focal epilepsies, in contrast to the Sherman study (2007) that linked inattentiveness with localization-related epilepsies.

Behavior Disorders as a Form of Epilepsy

Episodic hyperkinetic behavior may sometimes occur as a manifestation of epilepsy, but the diagnosis is often not clearly determined and "behavioral epilepsy" is controversial. A 4-year-old boy with benign partial epilepsy and hyperkinetic behavior between seizures is reported from Sapporo Medical University, Japan. Seizures consisted of a terrified expression, crouching, and rubbing his face on the floor. An EEG during a seizure in his sleep showed slow rhythms over the left hemisphere followed by depression of the voltage. Both the seizures and the hyperkinetic behavior responded to carbamazepine anticonvulsant therapy. The epilepsy was characterized as benign partial epilepsy with affective symptoms (Wakai et al., 1994). ADHD children with rolandic spikes in the EEG tend to exhibit more hyperactive-impulsive symptoms (ADHD-combined type) than inattention (ADD-inattentive type) (Hollmann ct al., 2003).

The association of an epileptiform EEG and a behavior disorder is sometimes considered to be coincidental (Okubo et al., 1994). However, if the behavioral symptoms are paroxysmal or appear in episodes, a trial of antiepileptic medication is justified.

Headache Disorders and ADHD

Classification of Headaches

According to the International Headache Society, International Classification of Headache Disorders-II (ICIID-II) 2004, *migraine* and *tension-type headache* are the two major types of primary headache. Cluster headache and other primary headaches occur mainly in adults. Other forms of headache in children are those secondary to head trauma (post-traumatic headache), benign intracranial hypertension, or intracranial tumor, substance-induced headache, cold-induced (ice-cream) headache, sinus-related headache, and diet-related headache. The following is the list of headaches in the ICHD-II classification:

1. Migraine
2. Tension-type headache
3. Cluster headache and other trigeminal cephalalgias
4. Other primary headaches (e.g., cough, exertional)
5. Headache attributed to head or neck trauma
6. Headache due to cranial or cervical vascular disorder
7. Headache due to non-vascular intracranial disorder
8. Headache due to a substance or its withdrawal
9. Headache attributed to infection
10. Headache attributed to disorder of homeostasis
11. Headache attributed to disorder of cranium, neck, eyes, ears, nose, sinuses, teeth, or mouth
12. Headache attributed to psychiatric disorder

Prevalence of Headache in Children

In children with ADHD, common headache precipitants include stress at school, irregular meals, and stimulant medications. A study of recurrent headaches diagnosed in 100 consecutive children in a pediatric neurology practice found 42% were migrainous in type and 58% nonmigrainous. Of the migrainous types, 27% were classical migraine (migraine with aura) and 15% common migraine (migraine without aura). Nonmigrainous headaches were of the tension type in 18%, tension associated with ADHD and learning disabilities in 21%, "epilepsy equivalents" in 18%, and in one, an intracranial arachnoid cyst. Boys were affected in 60% and girls in 40% of cases (Millichap, 1978).

Prevalence of migraine headaches in children varies in different studies, depending on the age and sex of the children, and the diagnostic criteria used in the definition of migraine. The average prevalence is 5%, or 1 in 20 school children.

In a random sample of the childhood population of the City of Aberdeen, Scotland, migraine was diagnosed by interview in 11%, more than twice the average prevalence quoted in previous pediatric studies (Abu-Arefeh and Russell, 1994). Tension headache occurred in 1%, and sinusitis in 0.2%. Under 12 years of age, boys suffered from migraine more frequently than girls, and over 12 years of age, girls predominated. Children with headache lost a mean of 8 days of school a year as compared to 3 days lost for control subjects.

In a population-based study of more than 1000 school children in Goteborg, Sweden, the prevalence of frequent headache increased with age and school grade, from 3% in second grade to 10% in third grade. The risk of frequent headache correlated with class size, increasing with larger classes. An increased prevalence of headache among girls in higher school grades was linked to possible hormonal changes and greater sensitivity to interpersonal conflicts and family stress (Carlsson, 1996).

In school age children living in an urban area of Finland, the prevalence of headache, including migraine, increased significantly between 1972 and 1992. School physicians recorded a history of migraine at the time of routine medical examinations of 7-year-old children in 1.9% in 1974 and 5.7% in 1992. The highest increases occurred among children exposed to social instability and stress (Sillanpaa and Anttila, 1996). Similar increases in the prevalence of migraine were reported in the 1980s among adults in the United States.

Classifications of Headache Diagnoses Compared

The distribution of the various types of headache is dependent on the definition of terms. In particular, the percentage of cases diagnosed as migraine without or with aura is modified according to the classification employed. In a cohort of 496 patients studied from 1992 to 2002 in a State University in Brazil, using the ICHD-I (1988) criteria, 11% of headache patients were diagnosed as migraine without aura and 5.2%, with aura. By ICHD-II (2004) diagnostic criteria, 28% had migraine without aura and 14.5%, with aura. When Standard diagnostic criteria (SD) were used, based on the intuitive clinical diagnosis of pediatric neurologists, 52% patients had migraine without aura and 20%, migraine with aura. In comparison, the respective frequencies of tension-type headache according to various classifications were very similar, at 19.6, 19 and 20.9%. The specificity for migraine diagnoses, without and with aura, was 100% for both ICHD-I and ICHD-II criteria. In contrast, the sensitivity for migraine diagnoses was relatively low, at 21% (without aura) and 27% (with aura) using ICHD-I-1988 criteria, and 53% (without aura) and 71% (with aura) for ICHD-II-2004 criteria (Lima et al., 2005). Sensitivities were improved to 98 and 97% for the two classifications when patients diagnosed as "migrainous disorder" or "probable migraine" were reevaluated according to diagnostic modifications and added to the migraine without and migraine with aura groups.

Diagnostic Modifications for Pediatric Migraine

International Classification of Headache Disorders (ICHD) criteria for the diagnosis of migraine include modifications for children and adolescents (IHS, 2004). These changes address the duration of the migraine episodes and the location of the headache (unilateral or bilateral) in migraine without aura. Migraine with aura is characterized by distinctive manifestations, and modifications are not required for pediatric patients. The ICHD-II–2004 duration of the migraine attack is changed from 4–72 h in adults to 2–48 h for children and adolescents under 15 years of age. If the minimum duration is reduced to 1 h or even one half hour, as in some standard diagnostic criteria, sensitivity is increased further (Maytal et al., 1997). Modifications of the International Headache Society (HIS) diagnostic criteria for pediatric migraine without aura are shown in Table 7.1.

Further modifications of the IHS criteria for pediatric migraine without aura are suggested following analysis of each headache characteristic listed in the ICHD-II (Hershey et al., 2005). When more relaxed criteria were employed in the review of diagnoses of 260 patients, sensitivity was improved to 84.4%. Modified criteria included bilateral headache, duration of 1–72 h, and nausea/or vomiting plus 2 of 5 other associated symptoms (photophobia, phonophobia, difficulty thinking, lightheadedness, or fatigue). The criteria moderate to severe, throbbing or pulsating pain, worsening or limiting physical activity were retained unchanged.

Childhood migraine compared to adult migraine has unique characteristics, including bilateral location, shorter duration, and difficulty with description of headache quality and associated symptoms. In children with ADHD, specificity of a migraine diagnosis is required to separate headaches of a tension or secondary type that would require different treatment.

If the above criteria (Table 7.2) are preceded within 1 h by visual hallucinations (bright lights or figures) or sensations of numbness or tingling lasting 5–60 minutes, the headaches are diagnosed as migraine with aura (classical migraine).

Table 7.2 Modified IHS criteria for pediatric migraine without aura

A. At least five attacks fulfilling B-D
B. Headache attack lasting 1–48 h[a]
C. Headache has at least two of the following:
    1. Unilateral or bilateral[a] location
    2. Pulsating quality
    3. Moderate to severe intensity
    4. Aggravation by routine physical activity
D. During headache, at least one of the following:
    1. Nausea and/or vomiting
    2. Photophobia and phonophobia

[a]Modifications proposed by Maytal et al. (1997) and Herrshey et al. (2005)

Migraine with aura is characterized by focal neurological symptoms that usually precede or sometimes accompany the headache. A premonitory phase, occurring hours or days before the headache, may be manifested by hyperactivity, hypoactivity, depression, craving for particular foods, or repetitive yawning.

A family history of migraine is a frequent finding that supports the diagnosis. Unlike tension headaches that often occur daily, migraine headaches recur at intervals of a week or usually longer. When symptoms are atypical, organic disease such as brain tumor must be ruled out.

Indications for MRI or CT in Children with Headaches

MRI or CT neuroimaging is recommended for:

- Headache with other signs of raised intracranial pressure
- Headache on awakening associated with vomiting
- Recurrent headache worsening in frequency and severity
- Headache with disturbance of consciousness and/or abnormal neurological signs
- Headache with seizure or focal EEG abnormality

The risk of an adverse reaction to CT contrast medium or to sedation necessary for MRI in young children must be weighed against the indications and potential benefits of the study.

Treatment of Headaches with ADHD

The following steps in the management of headaches associated with ADHD should be considered:

- Maintain headache diary
- Exclude specific causes of headache by history and examination, including infection (sinusitis) or raised intracranial pressure
- Relieve stress and tensions at school or at home
- Modify dosage or type of stimulant medication
- Investigate possible hypersensitivity to food items
- Medication for acute migraine attack

Family or individual psychological counseling may uncover reasons for stress-related headache. Larger doses of methylphenidate or amphetamines may need to be reduced or omitted, and alternative treatments considered. Dietary items known to precipitate headaches, such as chocolate, caffeine-containing sodas, hot dogs, aged cheeses, and dairy products, may need to be eliminated in sequence and for periods of up to 10 days (Millichap and Yee, 2003). Relief of symptoms should be followed by a challenge with the offending food or drink, to determine the significance of the apparent sensitivity. Long-term drug treatment for migraine in children is rarely necessary or advisable, provided the headache precipitants are uncovered and managed effectively.

Psychological Interventions in Management of Headaches

Psychologists at the *University of South Alabama, Mobile, AL* investigated the child's explanation of headache and description of the pain, as an aid to understanding the cause and best approach to management. A shift from emphasizing external methods of control to acknowledging self-control of headache occurs with increasing age. Treatments incorporating self-regulation of stress factors, such as biofeedback training, depend on the development of a child's awareness of effects of external events on the headaches. Attention and emphasis by the family on headache-free days can be a strong treatment reinforcer in children, focusing less attention on the symptom (Marcon and Labbe, 1990). Adding a developmental perspective to psychological interventions in the management of childhood headache is likely to increase treatment effectiveness.

Summary

Tics and Tourette syndrome, seizures, and headaches are occasional neurological complications of ADHD and its treatment. One in 4 school children with Tourette syndrome (TS) has ADHD, and stimulant therapy is the precipitant in 25% of comorbid cases. Of children treated with stimulants for ADHD by pediatric neurologists, 5% develop tics. TS is usually mild, and control with medication is required in less than half the cases encountered with ADHD. The association of TS with ADHD is a significant predictor of learning disabilities. A non-stimulant medication is preferred treatment for ADHD complicated by TS, and when possible, stimulants should be avoided or used in low dosage. Clonidine and guanfacine (Tenex®) are alternative therapies that may be indicated in resistant cases.

Epilepsy is frequently complicated by ADHD, and children with ADHD have a high incidence of subclinical epileptiform discharges in the EEG, especially centro-temporal spikes. Children with ADHD and abnormal EEG have an increased risk of seizures during treatment with stimulants. In children with comorbid epilepsy/ADHD whose seizures are controlled with antiepileptic medication, the introduction of stimulant therapy is safe and without risk of seizure recurrence.

Headache in children with ADHD may be precipitated by tension related to learning disability at school, irregular meals, and stimulant medications. Recommended interventions include a diagnostic evaluation, academic accommodations, a headache diary, elimination of food items known to trigger headache, and modification of dosage and type of ADHD medication.

References

Abu-Arefeh I, Russell G. Prevalence of headache and migraine in schoolchildren. *BMJ.* 1994;309:765–769.

Abwender DA, Como PG, Kurlan R, et al. School problems in Tourette's syndrome. *Arch Neurol.* 1996;53:509–511.

Baumgardner TL, Singer HS, Denckla MB, et al. Corpus callosum morphology in children with Tourette syndrome and attention deficit hyperactivity disorder. *Neurology.* 1996;47:477–482.

Biederman J, Melmed RD, Patel A, et al. A randomized, double-blind, placebo-controlled study of guanfacine extended release in children and adolescents with attention-deficit/hyperactivity disorder. *Pediatrics.* 2008;121:e73–e84.

Caine ED, et al. Tourette's syndrome in Monroe County school children. *Neurology.* 1988;38: 472–475.

Carlsson J. Prevalence of headache in schoolchildren: Relation to family and school factors. *Acta Paediatr.* 1996;85:692–696.

Carter AS, et al. A prospective longitudinal study of Gilles de la Tourette's syndrome. *J Am Acad Child Adolesc Psychiatry.* 1994;33:377–385.

Castaneda-Cabrero C, Lorenzo-Sanz G, Caro-Martinez E, et al. Electroencephalographic alterations in children with attention deficit hyperactivity disorder. *Rev Neurol*. 2003;37:904–908.

Chappell PB, Riddle MA, et al. Guanfacine treatment of comorbid attention-deficit hyperactivity disorder and Tourette's syndrome. *J Am Acad Child Adolesc Psychiatry*. 1995;34: 1140–1146.

Eapen V, Moriarty J, Robertson MM. Stimulus induced behaviors in Tourette's syndrome. *J Neurol Neurosurg Psychiatry*. 1994;57:853–855.

Eapen V, et al. Sex of parent transmission effect in Tourette's syndrome: evidence for earlier age at onset in maternally transmitted cases suggests a genomic imprinting effect. *Neurology*. 1997;48:934–937.

Fonseca LC, Tedrus GM, de Moraes C, de Vincente Machado A, de Almeida MP, de Oliveira DO. Epileptiform abnormalities and quantitative EEG in children with attention-deficit/hyperactivity disorder. *Arq Neuropsiquiatr*. 2008;66:462–467.

Gadow KD, Sverd J, Nolan EE, Sprafkion J, Schneider J. Immediate-release methylphenidate for ADHD in children with comorbid chronic multiple tic disorder. *J Am Acad Child Adolesc Psychiatry*. 2007;46:840–848.

Giedd JN, Rapoport JL, et al. Case study: acute basal ganglia enlargement and obsessive-compulsive symptoms in an adolescent boy. *J Am Acad Child Adolesc Psychiatry*. 1996;35:913–915.

Goodman & Gilman. *The Pharmacological Basis of Therapeutics*. 9th ed. New York: McGraw Hill; 1996.

Gross-Tsur V, et al. Epilepsy and attention deficit hyperactivity disorder: Is methylphenidate safe and effective? *J Pediatr*. 1997;130:670–674.

Guttmann E, et al. In: *Neurology*. Wilson SAK ed. Baltimore, MD: Williams and Wilkins, 1955; 1927: 1924.

Headache Classification Committee of the International Headache Society. The international classification of headache disorders-II. *Cephalalgia*. 2004;24(Suppl 1):137–149.

Hemmer SA, Pasternak JF, Zecker SG. Trommer BL Stimulant therapy and seizure risk in children with ADHD. *Pediatr Neurol*. 2001;24:99–102.

Hershey AD, Winner P, Kabbouche MA, et al. Use of the ICHD-II criteria in the diagnosis of pediatric migraine. *Headache*. 2005;45:1288–1297.

Hessen E, Lossius MI, Reinvang I, Gjerstad L. Influence of major antiepileptic drugs on attention, reaction time, and speed of information processing: results from a randomized, double-blind, placebo-controlled withdrawal study of seizure-free epilepsy patients receiving monotherapy. *Epilepsia*. 2006;47:2038–2045.

Holtmann M, Becker K, Kentner-Figura B, Schmidt MH. Increased frequency of rolandic spikes in ADHD children. *Epilepsia*. 2003;44:1241–1244.

Hughes JR, DeLeo AJ, Melyn MA. The electroencephalogram in attention deficit-hyperactivity disorder: emphasis on epileptiform discharges. *Epilepsy Behav*. 2000;1:271–277.

International Headache Society. The international classification of headache disorders. *Cephalalgia*. 2004;24(Suppl 1):1–160.

Kerbeshian J, et al. Comorbid Tourette's disorder and bipolar disorder: an etiologic perspective. *Am J Psychiatry*. 1995;152:1646–1651.

Kiesling LS, et al. Antineuronal antibodies in movement disorders. *Pediatrics*. 1993;92:39–43.

Kurlan R, et al. Transient tic disorder and the spectrum of Tourette's syndrome. *Arch Neurol*. 1988;45:1200–1201.

Lajonchere C, et al. Historical review of Gilles de la Tourette syndrome. *Arch Neurol*. 1996;53:567–574.

Lang A. Patient perception of tics and other movement disorders. *Neurology*. 1991;41:223–228.

Laporte N, Sebire G, Gillerot Y, Guerrini R, Ghariani S. Cognitive epilepsy: ADHD related to focal EEG discharges. *Pediatr Neurol*. 2002;27:307–311.

Lima MMF, Padula NAMR, Santos LCA, Oliveira LDB, Agapejev S, Padovani C. Critical analysis of the international classification of headache disorders diagnostic criteria (ICHD I-1988) and (ICHD II-2004), for migraine in children and adolescents. *Cephalalgia*. 2005;25: 1042–1047.

Lombroso PJ, et al. Exacerbation of Gilles de la Tourette's syndrome associated with thermal stress: a family study. *Neurology*. 1991;41:1984–1987.

Loring DW, Meador KJ. Cognitive side effects of antiepileptic drugs in children. *Neurology*. 2004;62:872–877.

Marcon RA, Labbe EE. Assessment and treatment of children's headaches from a developmental perspective. *Headache*. 1990;30:586–592.

Maytal J, Young M, Shechter A, Lipton RB. Pediatric migraine and the International Headache Society (HIS) criteria. *Neurology*. 1997;48:602–607.

Millichap JG ed. *Learning Disabilities and Related Disorders: Facts and Current Issues*. Chicago, IL: Year Book Med Publ; 1977.

Millichap JG. Recurrent headaches in 100 children. Electroencephalographic abnormalities and response to phenytoin (Dilantin). *Childs Brain*. 1978;4:95–104.

Millichap JG ed. *Progress in Pediatric Neurology II*. Chicago, IL: PNB Publishers; 1994: pp. 227–246.

Millichap JG ed. *Progress in Pediatric Neurology III*. Chicago, IL: PNB Publishers; 1997: pp. 257–258.

Millichap JG, Yee MM. The diet factor in pediatric and adolescent migraine. *Pediatr Neurol*. 2003;28:9–15.

Nordli DR Jr.. The management of epilepsy in children; cognitive and behavioral side effects. *Rev Neurol Dis*. 2004;1(Suppl 1):S4–S9.

Northram RS, Singer HS. Postencephalitic acquired Tourette-like syndrome in a child. *Neurology*. 1991;41:592–593.

Okubo Y, et al. Epileptiform EEG discharges in healthy children: Prevalence, emotional and behavioral correlates, and genetic influences. *Epilepsia*. 1994;35:832–841.

Parraga HC, Parraga MI, Harris DK. Tic exacerbation and precipitation during atomoxetine treatment in two children with attention-deficit hyperactivity disorder. *Int J Psychiatry Med*. 2007;37:415–424.

Piccirilli M, et al. Attention problems in epilepsy: Possible significance of the epileptogenic focus. *Epilepsia*. 1994;35:1091–1096.

Richer LP, Shevell MI, Rosenblatt BR. Epileptiform abnormalities in children with attention-deficit-hyperactivity disorder. *Pediatr Neurol*. 2002;26:125–129.

Schubert R. Attention deficit disorder and epilepsy. *Pediatr Neurol*. 2005;32:1–10.

Schuerholz LJ, et al. Learning disabilities in children with Tourette syndrome and ADHD. *Neurology*. 1996;46:958–965.

Schwabe MJ, Konkol RJ. Menstrual cycle-related fluctuations of tics in Tourette syndrome. *Pediatr Neurol*. 1992;8:43–46.

Sears J, Patel NC. Development of tics in a thirteen-year-old male following atomoxetine use. *CNS Spectr*. 2008;13:301–303.

Sherman EM, Slick DJ, Connolly MB, Eyrl KL. ADHD, neurological correlates and health-related quality of life in severe pediatric epilepsy. *Epilepsia*. 2007;48:1083–1091.

Sillanpaa M, Anttila P. Increasing prevalence of headache in 7-year-old schoolchildren. *Headache*. 1996;36:466–470.

Silvestri R, Gagliano A, Calarese T, et al. Ictal and interictal EEG abnormalities in ADHD children recorded over night by video-polysomnography. *Epilespy Res*. 2007;75:130–137.

Singer HS, Denckla MB, et al. Volumetric MRI changes in basal ganglia of children with Tourette's syndrome. *Neurology*. 1993;43:950–956.

Spencer T, Biederman J, et al. The relationship between tic disorders and Tourette's syndrome. *J Am Acad Child Adolesc Psychiatry*. 1995;34:1133–1139.

Tan M, Appleton R. Attention deficit and hyperactivity disorder, methylphenidate, and epilepsy. *Arch Dis Child*. 2005;90:57–59.

Wakai S, et al. Benign partial epilepsy with affective symptoms: Hyperkinetic behavior during interictal periods. *Epilepsia*. 1994;35:810–812.

Wilson SAK. *Neurology*. 2nd ed. Baltimore, MD: Williams and Wilkins; 1955.

Chapter 8
Methods of Management of ADHD

Several methods and disciplines are involved in the management of the child with ADHD. These include participation of the parents, teachers, psychologist, and physicians. The parents, and especially the mother, may be the first to draw attention to the problem, even in the preschool years. The teacher generally reports concerns about a child's inattention, hyperactivity, and impulsive behavior in kindergarten or first grade. The psychologist becomes involved either on referral from the teacher or after consultation with the physician. The pediatrician, pediatric neurologist, or child psychiatrist is usually consulted to confirm the diagnosis and to supervise the management of medical therapy.

Stimulant medications may have the most remarkable and prompt beneficial effects in the treatment of ADHD, but without family counseling, behavior modification, and remedial education, drugs alone will have only a partial and sometimes transitory value. The physician is in the ideal position to ensure that this so-called multimodal approach to the management of ADHD is followed, since the patient and parents will be seen at regular intervals for monitoring of medication effects and renewal of prescriptions. Reports from teachers, psychologist, and counselor should be made available to the physician at follow-up examinations.

American Academy of Pediatrics Clinical Practice Guidelines

Two sets of guidelines provide recommendations for the assessment and diagnosis of ADHD in school-aged children (AAP, 2000) and treatment of ADHD (AAP, 2001). The *Diagnosis Guideline* lists the following recommendations:

1. An evaluation for ADHD should be initiated in a child 6–12 years old who presents with inattention, hyperactivity, impulsivity, academic underachievement, or behavior problems;
2. The child should meet Diagnostic and Statistical Manual of Mental Disorders, 4th edition criteria for ADHD;
3. Evidence of ADHD should be obtained directly from parents or caregivers regarding the core symptoms of ADHD in various settings, duration of symptoms, and degree of functional impairment;

J.G. Millichap, *Attention Deficit Hyperactivity Disorder Handbook*,
DOI 10.1007/978-1-4419-1397-5_8, © Springer Science+Business Media, LLC 2010

4. Evidence of ADHD should be obtained directly from the classroom teacher;
5. Associated (coexisting) conditions should be assessed;
6. Other diagnostic tests may be indicated for associated learning disabilities or mental impairment.

The AAP *Treatment Guideline* recommends the following:

1. The clinician should recognize ADHD as a chronic condition;
2. Specify target outcomes to guide management;
3. Recommend stimulant medication and/or behavior therapy to improve target outcomes;
4. When the selected management has not met target outcomes, clinicians should evaluate the original diagnosis, use of appropriate treatments, and presence of coexisting conditions;
5. Conduct periodic monitoring of the effects of treatment by office visit every 3–6 months;
6. If one stimulant does not work at the highest feasible dose, another should be recommended.

Studies of adherence to the AAP Guidelines have shown an overall response rate of 60%, but only 26% reported routine use of all diagnostic components. Some clinicians included diagnostic modalities not recommended for routine evaluations – continuous performance testing, neuroimaging, and laboratory tests (e.g., thyroid, lead, or iron testing). The majority (66.6%) of respondents reported routine use of medications and 81% titrated the dose of medication in the first month; 53% reported routine follow-up visits, 3–4 times per year. A majority of clinicians (53%) also recommended behavioral therapy. Half of respondents reported that insurers limited coverage for assessment and treatment of ADHD, and 32% reported poor access to mental health services in the community (Rushton et al., 2004).

Some communities have developed a protocol to ensure collaboration between educators and physicians (Foy and Earis, 2005). School personnel are asked to provide the following; (a) vision and hearing screening; (b) teacher behavior rating scales (e.g., Vanderbilt, Conner, or Achenbach); (c) speech/language evaluation when indicated; (d) screening intelligence and achievement testing; (e) full intelligence testing when indicated; (f) consider need for an individualized education plan (IEP, special education) or 504 plan with classroom accommodations; and (g) use communication forms to share medication responses.

The AAP Committees on Quality Improvement and ADHD reviewed the current literature for the purpose of developing an evidence-based clinical practice guideline for the treatment of the school-aged child with ADHD (Brown et al., 2005). The evidence strongly supports the use of stimulant medications for treating the core symptoms and, to a lesser degree, for improving functioning of children with ADHD. Behavior therapy alone has only limited effect on symptoms or functioning of children with ADHD. In combination with medication, behavior therapy may improve functioning and may decrease the amount of stimulant medication needed. Comparison of stimulants (methylphenidate and amphetamines) shows no significant difference in effectiveness.

Guidelines are not intended as a sole source of guidance for the treatment of children with ADHD. They are designed to assist the primary care clinician by providing a framework for decision-making. They are not intended to replace clinical judgment or to establish a protocol for all children with ADHD and may not provide the only appropriate approach to this problem (AAP, 2001).

Principal Forms of Therapy of ADHD

A single approach to the management of ADHD is never completely satisfactory, despite the dramatic early benefits of stimulant therapy. In addition to medications that are discussed more fully in the next chapter, important therapeutic regimens include the following:

- Psychological and psychosocial intervention
- Parent and family counseling
- Behavior modification and/or child counseling
- Remedial education and learning accommodations

The optimal order of introduction of these various methods of management is somewhat controversial. Some psychologists favor initial psychosocial intervention and behavior modification management, whereas physicians often prefer to introduce medication early as an essential aid to education and academic success.

Roles of the Psychologist and Psychiatrist in the Management of the Child with ADHD

The psychologist provides testing, diagnosis, and/or counseling in group or individual sessions, and advises on class placement, behavior management, and appropriate academic accommodations. The psychiatrist diagnoses and treats with medications and psychotherapy. Some university-based psychiatrists are psychopharmacologists, specializing in the research and trials of medications for ADHD and comorbid disorders.

Psychologist s specialize as educational or clinical psychologists, providing testing and/or therapy. Some are trained to provide both types of services. A parent may consult a psychologist about symptoms of ADHD or a learning problem as a first resort or on the advice of the physician or teacher. At some point, a child who is having learning or behavioral problems will need the services of a psychologist These may be provided through the school or mental health system or privately.

The psychological effects of a disabled child on family functioning, peer relationships, and methods of counseling and training of families of children with ADHD are discussed by Barkley (1997) and Millichap (1984).

Physician's Role in Helping the Parents to Understand and Deal with the Problem of ADHD

Since the medical evidence supports a neurobiological or organic basis for ADHD, the major responsibility for the problem has been shifted from the parents to the child's brain and a neurochemical or structural brain deficit. The claim by sociologists and others that ADHD represents a "deviant behavior," largely under the control of the child and parent–child relationship, has been discounted by neurological research. The "medicalization" of ADHD and its treatment as an "illness" has been justified by the results of scientific studies.

The physician explains the factors known to underlie the symptoms of ADHD and orders tests to rule out specific causes as appropriate. While the physician is responsible for the diagnosis and medical management, the parents need to understand the influence of child–family interaction and remedial education on the success of treatment interventions. The parents have an equal responsibility to become educated in their role in the management of the child in the home. Parental conflict and environmental family adversity will exacerbate the symptoms of ADHD and diminish the effectiveness of medical treatment (Millichap, 1975).

Useful Advice for Parents in Management of ADHD

To live with a hyperactive child demands patience and understanding of parents, siblings, and neighbors. The following suggestions for parents may be found helpful:

- Avoid repetition of "no" and "don't."
- Use praise whenever appropriate and emphasize successful activities to build self-confidence and self-esteem.
- Find an academic or sports interest that motivates a child and encourage and support it.
- Speak quietly and slowly.
- Present tasks or errands, one at a time.
- Use written or picture cues to reinforce verbal requests or explanations.
- Encourage a structured, calm routine for homework, mealtimes, playtime, and bedtime.
- Avoid formal meals in restaurants if they lead to disruption and argument.
- Encourage less boisterous playmates and avoid noisy activities.
- Obtain the help of a family counselor or psychologist, especially if the ADHD is complicated by oppositional defiant or conduct disorder.

Of all these parental interventions, perhaps the emphasis on motivation is the most important.

Motivational Techniques Emphasized in Parent Counseling and Training Sessions

Parents often ask why their child can focus on an activity such as Nintendo or a favorite television program while exhibiting distractibility and inattentiveness in school. The answer is related to the nature of attention and the influence of environmental demands and distractions.

The learning process may be classified in four categories:

1. *goal-awareness*,
2. *vigilance*,
3. *selectivity*, and
4. *tenacity*.

The child with ADHD is usually hypervigilant, but has deficits in selection and sustaining attention (Rosenberger, 1991). The discrimination of essential from unessential stimuli is impaired. Attention can be redirected by situational demands and goal-awareness or motivation.

Parents may encourage the child to pursue appropriate interests by finding motivational activities and providing support and praise. Biographies of famous people who have overcome adversity to succeed in their chosen field of endeavor are excellent motivational tools (Millichap and Millichap, 1986).

Winston Spencer Churchill, who saved England from the tyranny of Hitler's Germany by his superior leadership and oratory, and later wrote a best-selling History of the British Empire, had symptoms of ADHD, a speech impediment and learning disability as a child (Churchill, 1930). In his autobiography, *My Early Life*, Churchill wrote: "I was on the whole considerably discouraged by my school days." "It is not pleasant to feel oneself so completely outclassed and left behind at the very beginning of the race." He was surprised on leaving school to hear his teacher predict, "with a confidence for which I could see no foundation, that I should be able to make my way all right." "I have always been very grateful to him for this remark."

A simple word of praise or note of confidence from a teacher makes its mark for life in a child with academic problems. Churchill did indeed make his way all right. He became Prime Minister of Great Britain and a World leader. Like Churchill, several famous people have been reported to suffer from learning disabilities during childhood. Thomas Edison, Albert Einstein, President Woodrow Wilson, and Governor Nelson Rockefeller are among those listed as dyslexic, yet their names are indelibly written in the papers of history.

In the book on dyslexia (Millichap and Millichap, 1986), Nancy Millichap refers to articles on the childhood of Thomas Edison and other historical figures. Thomas Edison, inventor, was diagnosed as mentally ill by his teacher, his father thought he was stupid, he never learned to spell, and up to the time of his manhood his grammar was appalling. Albert Einstein, physicist and Nobel Prize winner, did not talk until he was four nor read until nine. Einstein was considered to be backward by his teachers and his father. Woodrow Wilson, President of the United States, did not learn his letters until he was nine or learn to read until he was eleven. Nelson A. Rockefeller, the former governor of New York State and vice-president of the United States, in an article written in the TV Guide, 1976, titled "Don't Accept Anyone's Verdict That You are Lazy, Stupid, or Retarded," recalled his difficulties as a dyslexic boy. In his day, classes and teachers for reading-disabled children were not available. Nowadays, with our current understanding of dyslexia and other learning disabilities, the burden of a child's academic problems should be lighter and prospects brighter.

The Child's Involvement in Management of ADHD

The physician, parent, and teacher each has a role in counseling the child with ADHD. Specialized psychological or psychiatric counseling is required in patients with behavior, mood or anxiety disorders, resistant to more simple measures. Behavior modification therapy employing rewards may be helpful as an adjunct to medical treatment.

The physician explains the nature of the disorder and purpose of medications. Methylphenidate (Ritalin®) is recommended as an aid to education, to help focus and lessen distractibility, not primarily to modify behavior. Although the practice of interrupting therapy is debatable, medicines may be omitted at weekends and on vacations. Exceptions to drug holidays include the child engaged in learning or homework assignments, and impulsive behavior that poses a danger to the safety and well-being.

Parents should praise success, ignore failure, and avoid excessive or harsh criticism, but tolerance should be tempered with appropriate and consistent discipline. Teachers, with the help of the psychologist, explain the nature of the learning problem, emphasizing the strengths and showing how weaknesses may be corrected by training. A positive attitude of parents, teachers, and all professionals is the key to success.

Behavior Modification Therapy: Methods and Results

Behavior modification is a systematic form of environmental structuring, based on the hypothesis that behavior is governed by either pleasurable or denied gratification. It is assumed that a child will modify behavior to obtain rewards and to avoid restrictions, denials, or reprimands.

A system of rewards, denials, or reprimands is established and explained fully to the child and all members of the family. Both parents in the home and teachers in the classroom should be involved. Good or desirable behavior is rewarded and positively reinforced, and bad or undesirable behavior is negatively reinforced. Positive reinforcements are usually preferred and emphasized although immediate reprimands may be necessary as a more intense behavioral intervention. Tokens used as positive reinforcement are given to the child and exchanged for goods or services according to a schedule of rates and values. Time outs in a quiet room and denial or restriction of television viewing time are examples of negative reinforcements and the consequences of unacceptable behavior.

Classroom reinforcers include individualized attention, immediate and frequent praise for good work, and responsibility and rewards for special tasks. If necessary, reprimands should be administered immediately and not delayed. An Emory University study of ADHD children's responses to behavioral intervention alone and in combination with stimulant medication showed that immediate classroom teacher reprimands can achieve results comparable to those of stimulants. However, such behavioral interventions are labor intensive and not accessible to most children with ADHD. Furthermore, for some children medication will obviate the need for intensive behavioral intervention (Abramowitz et al., 1992).

Behavior modification requires time, patience, and some compulsiveness on the part of the parents, teachers, and therapists. If the system is to be applied uniformly and consistently over an extended period, the detailed explanations necessary are usually outside the scope of most physicians in practice. Parents interested in the method should obtain professional assistance through the local community mental health center or a private consulting psychologist or psychiatrist (Dulcan, 1994).

In practice, behavior modification alone is rarely successful, but in combination with medication it can be of value. In children with ADHD complicated by ODD or CD, individual counseling with a psychologist or social worker is usually required.

The Role of the Teacher and School System in the Management of ADHD

The teacher is often the first person to recognize a child's inattention, hyperactivity and impulsiveness, and to suspect a diagnosis of ADHD. After discussion with the parents, the teacher may complete ADHD and behavioral questionnaires, such as the Conner, McCarney, Quay and Peterson, or Vanderbilt Rating Scales. On the basis of a child's inability to function satisfactorily in the normal classroom and the results of the questionnaires, further testing by a school psychologist or learning disability teacher may be implemented. A consultation with the child's pediatrician or with a pediatric neurologist will be suggested.

The appropriate accommodations in class placement and school curriculum should be made after parent–teacher conferences are completed. Learning disabilities uncovered by psychological tests should be remedied by special methods of education. The educational rights of children with ADD are protected by federal law.

Federal Laws Relating to Educational Rights of Children with ADHD

Two federal laws guarantee appropriate education for children with ADHD enrolled in public schools or private schools receiving federal funds. These are the *Individuals with Disabilities Act (IDEA)* and *Section 504 of the Rehabilitation Act of 1973*. The Department of Education, in a "Policy Clarification Memorandum," dated September 16, 1991, states that students with ADD are eligible for special education and related services under Part B of the IDEA, solely on the basis of their ADD when it significantly impairs educational performance or learning.

As with other disabilities included under the IDEA, it must be established that the ADD has significant negative impact on a child's educational performance. A multidisciplinary team evaluation may be required to determine whether special education and/or related services are needed. An Individual Educational Program (IEP) is arranged for children in need of resource room aide or training.

While the IDEA requires a child with ADD to have a learning problem for eligibility for special services, Section 504 covers children with behavior problems such as hyperactivity, not complicated by learning disabilities.

The Americans with Disabilities Act (ADA), 1990, provides additional legal requirements that cover children with ADD attending public schools and non-religious private schools. A local CHADD (Children and Adults with Attention Deficit Disorders) chapter will provide parents with information if help is needed in obtaining special educational services.

Classroom Accommodations for Children with ADHD and Learning Disorders

The Federal Government Department of Education suggests classroom accommodations and remedial education that include the following examples:

- Structured learning environment
- Individualized homework assignments
- Written as well as verbal instructions
- Extended time for tests
- Access to tape recorders and computers
- Behavior modification techniques

The parent should meet with the teacher in order to discuss and implement the recommended changes in a child's curriculum. The parent is usually involved in this "individual educational plan or program (IEP)."

Public School Special Education Placements for Children with ADHD

The various special education programs are graded according to the severity and type of the child's learning and/or behavior disorder, from mild to severe, as follows:

1. Regular classroom plus part-time tutoring,
2. Regular classroom plus part-time resource room, 1/2–2 h daily.
3. Part-time learning disability class plus resource room and mainstreaming or integration into regular class for certain subjects.
4. Full-time learning disability (LD) or behavior disorder (ED) class.
5. Full-time "educable mentally disabled" class (intended for children with an IQ of 60–80 and not classified as ADHD or LD).

The advantages of the resource room and the learning disability class are the small size, which allows for more individual attention, and staffing by teachers with special qualification in the field of learning disorders. The disadvantage of such classes is the stigma of labeling and segregating the child from peers at an early age. However, if the purpose is explained to the child individually and to the class and parents, the special education is soon accepted when academic successes result.

Professional Support Services in Public Schools

Specialized support services made available to children with ADHD attending public schools include the following:

- *School psychologist.* The psychologist is called upon to perform individual intelligence, perception, and reading tests if a child is thought to have a learning problem, and to evaluate social-emotional factors underlying behavior disorders. The *psychological evaluation* administered individually is different from the *achievement tests* (Iowa, Stanford, or California) that are administered to a group by the classroom or learning disability teacher at more frequent intervals. Parents are often confused about the functions and tests performed by the psychologist and the LD teacher.
- *Social worker.* The school social worker may provide counseling services for children with behavioral problems, and emotional support and reassurance for those dealing with issues such as divorce or peer pressures.
- *School nurse.* The school nurse often takes the responsibility for handing out medications at lunchtime, for reporting any side effects, and supervises records of required immunizations, and vision and hearing tests.
- *Remedial reading teacher.* Children with dyslexia or lesser degrees of reading difficulty can be referred to the reading specialist for individual or group instruction and training.
- *Speech pathologist.* Speech and language evaluations are performed by the school staff, if a child's understanding and/or expressive language abilities are delayed. The speech pathologist also provides therapy individually or in groups.
- *School guidance counselor.* Guidance counselors are available particularly in high schools. They assist students with selection of classes, careers, and colleges. In lower grades a guidance counselor may help with tutors and decisions regarding grade placement or special schools.

- *Occupational therapist.* Occupational therapy (OT) sessions are sometimes advised for children with ADHD complicated by motor incoordination. OT will often help in facilitating gross coordination, permitting children to participate in group physical activities.

Indications for a Private or Therapeutic School Education for Children with ADHD

Private educational facilities for children with ADHD are either day schools or boarding schools. The private day school or therapeutic school may be essential when the public school district is unable to provide appropriate special educational services. The boarding school may be the ideal placement for the child who requires special services in a well-structured environment on a 24-h basis.

Children with both learning and language disorders may not show the expected rate of progress in regular public school placements and may require more intensive and individualized teaching programs. The small teacher–pupil ratio in private schools is an advantage, but the fees necessary to provide this optimal placement are often prohibitive.

Role of the Tutor in the Education of the Child with ADHD

Individual tutoring is the most flexible and least conspicuous method of providing special education. In addition to supplementing school instruction, the experienced tutor will often assume the role of counselor and advisor, bolstering self-confidence and allaying a child's anxieties about school performance. When a tutor is recommended, the choice should be made in consultation with the regular classroom teacher if possible. This allows continuity between the work in the classroom and homework.

Resource Groups and Associations Available to Parents for Information on ADHD and Learning Disabilities

A number of national and local resource groups provide information on ADHD for parents on request. The web site address for ADHD is as follows:

http://www.healthguide.com/adhd/

CHADD, the organization for Children and Adults with Attention Deficit Disorders, provides information and support for parents, including suggestions on parent training, medical management, and educational rights for children with ADD. They also provide information for teachers, and a review of controversial alternative treatments. Each local chapter has regular evening meetings and frequent guest speakers who are experts in various aspects of ADHD. CHADD national office address is as follows:

CHADD
8181 Professional Place, Suite 150
Landover, MD 20785
Tel: 800-233-4050; Fax: 301-306-7090
Web site: http://www.help4adhd.org

LDAA, the Learning Disabilities Association of America, arranges educational symposia on ADHD and learning disabilities, with invited speakers and research presentations. They also publish camp and college directories suited to young people with LD. Their address is as follows:

LDAA
4156 Library Road
Pittsburgh, PA 15234
Tel: 412-341-1515; Fax: 412-344-0224
Web site: http://www.ldaamerica.org

ADDA, National Attention Deficit Disorder Association:

15000 Commerce Pkwy, Suite C, Mount Laurel, NJ 08054
Tel: 856-439-9099; Fax: 856-439-0525
Web site: http://www.add.org
e-mail: adda@add.org

NATIONAL CENTER FOR LEARNING DISABILITIES

381 Park Avenue South, Suite 1401
New York, NY 10016 E-mail:help@ncld.org
Tel: 212-545-7510; Fax: 212-545-9665

INTERNATIONAL DYSLEXIA ASSOCIATION, Formerly, Orton Dyslexia Society provides information on the study, treatment, and prevention of dyslexia.

40 York Road, Suite 400
Towson, MD 21204
Tel: 800-222-3123
Fax: 410-321-5069
E-mail: info@interdys.org
http://www.interdys.org/index.jsp

KENNEDY KRIEGER INSTITUTE CENTER FOR DEVELOPMENT AND LEARNING

707 North Broadway
Baltimore, MD 21205
Tel: 888-554-2080
Fax: 443-923-9405
E-mail: info@kennedykrieger.org
http://www.kennedykrieger.org

Summary

Management of ADHD is multimodal and involves the participation of parent, teacher, psychologist, and physician. The American Academy of Pediatrics has issued guidelines with recommendations for assessment, diagnosis, and treatment of ADHD. They provide a framework for decision-making. They are not intended to replace clinical judgment or to establish a protocol for all children with ADHD. In addition to medication, principal forms of therapy include psychological and psychosocial intervention, parent and family counseling, behavior modification, and remedial education and learning accommodations.

Evidence strongly supports the use of stimulant medications for treating the core symptoms and for improving functioning of children with ADHD. Behavior modification alone has only limited effect on symptoms or functioning but in combination with medication, behavior therapy may improve functioning and may decrease the amount of stimulant medication needed. Methylphenidate and amphetamine stimulants are equally effective, when monitored frequently, using schoolteacher in addition to parent reports of progress.

References

Abramowitz AJ, Dulcan MK, et al. ADHD children's responses to stimulant medication and two intensities of a behavioral intervention. *Behav Modif.* 1992;16:193–203.

American Academy of Pediatrics. Clinical practice guideline: diagnosis and evaluation of the child with attention-deficit/hyperactivity disorder. *Pediatrics.* 2000;105:1158–1170.

American Academy of Pediatrics. Clinical practice guideline: treatment of the school-aged child with attention-deficit/hyperactivity disorder. *Pediatrics.* 2001;108:1033–1044.

Barkley RA. *Attention-Deficit Hyperactivity Disorder: A Handbook for Diagnosis and Treatment* 3rd ed. New York: Guildford Press; 1997.

Brown RT, Amier RW, Freeman WS, et al; American Academy of Pediatrics Committee on Quality Improvement; American Academy of Pediatrics Subcommittee on Attention-Deficit/Hyperactivity Disorder. Treatment of attention-deficit/hyperactivity disorder: overview of the evidence. *Pediatrics.* 2005;115:e749–e757.

Churchill WS. *My Early Life. A Roving Commission.* New York: Charles Scribner's Sons; 1930.

Dulcan MK. Treatment of children and adolescents. In: Hales RE, Yodofsky SC, Talbott JA eds. *The American Psychiatric Press Textbook of Psychiatry.* 2nd ed. Washington, DC: American Psychiatric Press; 1994:1209–1250.

Foy JM, Earis MF. A process for developing community consensus regarding the diagnosis and management of attention-deficit/hyperactivity disorder. *Pediatrics*. 2005;115:e97–e104.

Millichap JG. *The Hyperactive Child with Minimal Brain Dysfunction. Questions and Answers*. Chicago, IL: Year Book Medical Publishers; 1975.

Millichap MG. The Effects of the Developmentally Disabled Child on the Family. Roosevelt University, Masters Degree Thesis, Chicago, 1984.

Millichap NM. Dyslexia: Theories of Causation and Methods of Management, an Historical Perspective. Loyola University of Chicago, Masters Degree Thesis, 1986.

Millichap NM, Millichap JG. *Dyslexia: As the Educator and Neurologist Read It*. Springfield, IL: Charles C Thomas; 1986.

Rosenberger PB. Attention deficit. *Pediatr Neurol*. 1991;7:397–405.

Rushton JL, Fant KE, Clark SJ. Use of practice guidelines in the primary care of children with attention-deficit/hyperactivity disorder. *Pediatrics*. 2004;114:e–23.

Chapter 9
Medications for ADHD

Medications, especially central nervous system stimulants, are an important part of treatment of ADHD. The use of stimulants for the treatment of hyperactive behavior in children was first described in 1937, beginning with amphetamines. Controlled trials of methylphenidate (Ritalin®) in the 1960s demonstrated significant benefits without serious side effects. In addition to a lessening of motor activity, focus and attention were increased and schoolwork, grades, and social behavior were improved (Conners and Eisenberg, 1963). In small to moderate doses, methylphenidate benefits learning without impairing creative or flexible thinking. The value of stimulant medication in the management of ADHD has withstood the test of time.

Ongoing research has provided answers to many of the parents' concerns, and has confirmed the effectiveness and safety of the long-term use of medication.

Stimulant Medications Recommended for Treatment of ADHD

Lists of central nervous stimulant medications available for treatment of ADHD are shown in Tables 9.1 and 9.2. Ritalin® or its generic form, methylphenidate, is the prototype central nervous stimulant for the treatment of ADHD. Ritalin-SR and Concerta™ are extended-release, long-acting preparations of methylphenidate. The earliest reported use of stimulant medications for hyperactive children is usually credited to Bradley (1937), who first employed Benzedrine (D,L-amphetamine) and later, in 1950, Dexedrine (D-amphetamine). Benzedrine is no longer available, and Dexedrine is largely replaced by Adderall®, a mixture of amphetamines, that appears to have properties superior to D-amphetamine alone. Lisdexamfetamine, a new amphetamine marketed under the brand name, Vyvanse®, has an onset of action slower than that of Dexedrine, with peak effect at 2.5 h and duration of action up to 12 h. Cylert® (pemoline) is another long-acting stimulant, but because of reported liver toxicity, it is no longer prescribed.

Differences in potency of the brand, trade preparation, Ritalin®, and the generic form, methylphenidate, are occasionally encountered in practice. The substitution of the Ritalin brand for the generic preparation may result in a change in effectiveness. A lack of response to generic methylphenidate should prompt a trial of the brand

J.G. Millichap, *Attention Deficit Hyperactivity Disorder Handbook*,
DOI 10.1007/978-1-4419-1397-5_9, © Springer Science+Business Media, LLC 2010

Table 9.1 Methylphenidate formulations of stimulant medication

Brand name	Strengths (mg)	Release	Peak (h)	Duration (h)
Short-acting				
Ritalin	5, 10, 20	Fast	1–2	3–4
Methylin	5, 10, 20 chewable	Fast	1–2	3–4
	2.5, 5, 10 solution	Fast	1–2	3–4
Focalin[a]	2.5, 5, 10	Fast	1–2	3–6
Intermediate-acting				
Ritalin SR	20	Slower	4–5	7–8
Methylin ER	10, 20	Slower	4–5	7–8
Metadate ER	10, 20	Slower	4–5	7–8
Extended release				
Ritalin LA	10, 20, 30, 40	Biphasic	1–3, 5–8	8–10
			50% am	50% later
Metadate CD	10, 20, 30, 40, 50, 60	Biphasic	1–2, 4–5	10–12
			30% am	70% later
Focalin XR	5, 10, 15, 20	Biphasic	1–2, 6–7	10–12
Concerta	18, 27, 36, 54	Biphasic	1–2, 6–8	10–12
Daytrana patch	10, 15, 20, 30	Slow	Plateau	9–10

[a]Dexmethylphenidate

Table 9.2 Dextroamphetamine formulations of stimulant medication

Brand name	Strengths (mg)	Release	Peak (h)	Duration (h)
Short-acting				
Dexedrine	5, 10	Fast	2–3	5–6
Dextrostat	10	Fast	2–3	5–6
Intermediate-acting				
Adderall*	10, 12.5, 15, 20, 30	Variable	2–3	5–7
Dexedrine spans	5, 10, 15	Long	7–8	12
Extended release				
Adderall XR[a]	5, 10, 15, 20, 25, 30	Long	7–8	12
Vyvanse[b]	20, 30, 40, 50, 60, 70	Slow	3–4	12

[a]Dextro- and levo-amphetamines
[b]Lisdexamfetamine

Ritalin before accepting failure of stimulant therapy. In subsequent references to trials of stimulant medications, the brand or the generic name will be listed depending on which form was prescribed.

Paradoxical Calming Effect of Stimulant Medications

The primary function of a psychostimulant medication is to increase focus and alertness. Structurally, the amphetamines resemble neurotransmitters, catecholamines that facilitate the passage of impulses from one nerve cell to another. They are thought to increase catecholamine activity at neuronal synapses, leading to a buildup of the neurotransmitters, norepinephrine and dopamine, and at higher doses, serotonin. The D-isomer has a greater effect on dopaminergic transmission and is a more potent stimulant than the L-isomer. Methylphenidate is structurally similar to amphetamines and a dopamine and catecholamine reuptake inhibitor. It increases the concentration of neurotransmitters at the synaptic cleft, but enhancement of serotonin transmission by methylphenidate is less than with amphetamines.

The brain has both excitatory and inhibitory motor pathways that are influenced by the neurochemical transmitters. A deficiency in neurotransmitters could weaken inhibition and permit excessive motor activity. In theory, children with ADHD are lacking in brain dopamine and norepinephrine. The so-called paradoxical calming effect of psychostimulants may be related to an increase and correction in the levels of these neurotransmitter chemicals in the brain, restoring the function of inhibitory pathways. These chemical effects are thought to normalize motor activity while still preserving and heightening the degree of alertness.

The metabolic pathways in the formation of catecholamines and the effects of amphetamines are as follows:

TYROSINE>DOPA>DOPAMINE>NOREPINEPHRINE

Enzymes and cofactors, including pyridoxal phosphate and ascorbate, are involved in these pathways. Catecholamines are concentrated in storage vesicles within nerve terminals. Amphetamines displace catecholamines from the storage vesicles, resulting in leakage of neurotransmitters from the nerve terminals.

An alternative or supplement to the neurochemical explanation is based on the neuroanatomical location of the action of psychostimulants and their effect on the frontal lobe, an area with an inhibitory influence on motor activity.

Specific Benefits of Stimulant Medication in ADHD

In addition to a more focused behavior, the child is less distractible, has a longer attention span and is less active and impulsive. Visual perception, eye–hand coordination, drawing and handwriting are improved, schoolwork is more organized, and achievement of better grades is facilitated.

In one of the earliest controlled studies of the effectiveness of Ritalin®, conducted at *Children's Memorial Hospital, NWU, Chicago*, 68% of 30 children with ADHD were benefited during a 3-week trial period. Neuropsychological tests showed improvements in intelligence, visual memory, and eye–hand coordination (Millichap et al., 1968). A later review of the literature, and reports of a total of 337 children in seven different trials of Ritalin, showed that an average of 83% improved (Millichap, 1973).

Subsequent reports of trials of methylphenidate (MPH) and other central nervous stimulants, involving close to 5000 children, have continued to demonstrate a positive response in 70–80% of the subjects. Hyperactive behavior, self-esteem, learning, and social and family functioning are improved. Effects of MPH on comorbid oppositional and conduct disorders are varied, with some investigators reporting a lack of response (Spencer et al., 1996), while others noting an improvement in the teacher conduct ratings (DuPaul 1993). In general, MPH has a higher frequency of positive effects on ADHD than on comorbid oppositional and conduct disorders. Children who do not respond to medication require a greater emphasis on behavior modification and parent-family counseling (Abramowitz et al., 1992).

ADHD Patients Most Likely to Respond to Stimulant Medication

Children who are most active, impulsive, and distractible are most likely to benefit from methylphenidate (MPH) treatment. These predictors of response to MPH were reported in Millichap (1973) and confirmed in subsequent studies in Barkley et al. (1991) and Handen et al. (1994)). Although MPH may be indicated in a child with ADD without hyperactivity and impulsivity, a response is more likely when the inattentive child is also hyperactive.

The clinical judgment of the severity of ADHD and improvement observed after a single dose of MPH are useful predictors of a beneficial long-term response. Factors predictive of response to MPH were examined in 46 children with ADHD, treated at the University of Utrecht, The Netherlands (Buitelaar et al., 1995). MPH normalized behavior at school in one half the children and behavior at home in one third. Predictors of response to MPH included a high intelligence quotient, severe inattention, and absence of anxiety. Positive behavioral changes, measured by the Abbreviated Conners' Rating Scales after a single 10 mg dose of MPH, were predictive of continued improvements after 4 weeks of treatment.

Creativity and Flexibility of Thinking During Treatment with Methylphenidate

Some parents are concerned that a medication given to help focusing ability and control impulsivity may at the same time reduce creativity and flexibility of a child's thinking. Researchers investigating effects on creativity, measured by the Torrance nonverbal thinking test, found that methylphenidate (MPH) had no adverse effects on creative thinking in 19 boys with ADHD (Funk et al., 1993). Control of impulsivity is independent of creativity. Furthermore, flexibility of thinking and speed and accuracy of processing information were improved in studies using acute, single MPH doses of 0.3 and 0.6 mg (Douglas et al., 1995). In small to moderate doses, MPH does not impair a child's creativity and flexibility of thinking.

Relation of the Dose of Methylphenidate to the Response of ADHD Symptoms

The response to methylphenidate (MPH) is related to the dose, especially for tasks requiring attention. Cognitive performance and learning ability are improved by lower doses (0.3 mg/kg) whereas higher doses (1.0 mg/kg) may impair learning but improve social behavior, according to one report (Sprague and Sleator, 1977). A later study found that the beneficial effects of MPH on academic performance did not vary with dosage, but behavioral improvements were more prolonged with the larger dose (Tannock et al., 1989). The lower dose (0.3 mg/kg), taken in the morning, produced both academic and behavioral improvements that were no longer present in the afternoon. A higher morning dose (1.0 mg/kg) was followed by improvements in behavior that were sustained, and academic improvements that disappeared, by the afternoon. Side effects involving an increase in pulse rate and blood pressure were observed only with the larger dose.

More recent studies investigated the effects of MPH at four different dose levels, 5, 10, 15, and 20 mg (Rapport et al., 1994). The effects on classroom functioning, including on-task attention, assignment completion, and teacher ratings, were related to the dose of MPH. Accuracy of work was increased at all dose levels, and task completion was significantly greater at single doses above 5 mg. In children failing to respond to low dose MPH, focus of attention was responsive to dose increments, whereas behavior and academic achievement were not improved by larger doses.

These well-controlled research studies indicate that smaller doses of MPH will benefit both academic performance and behavior and are generally preferable to a single larger dose, but the action is short lived and the dose must be repeated to sustain effectiveness. In attempting to determine an optimal dose for each individual child, the duration of action on academic, cognitive, and behavioral performance must be evaluated.

At the Scottish Rite Children's Medical Center, Atlanta, GA, the effects on attention and learning of two different doses (0.3 and 0.8 mg/kg) of methylphenidate (MPH) were evaluated in 23 children, aged 7–11 years, with ADHD. An attention continuous performance task was improved with the low dose MPH, and impulsivity measured by the number of commission errors was reduced. On nonverbal learning and memory tasks, the easy level of task performance was improved equally with either dose of MPH, whereas the hard task was performed better only with the high dose (O'Toole et al., 1997).

Attention and impulsivity are benefited by low doses of MPH, but higher doses may be required to improve retention and recall of complex nonverbal information. Cognitive function and behavior are sensitive to stimulant medication, but doses must be individualized and titrated for each patient.

MPH is generally administered two or three times a day, after breakfast, at lunchtime at school, and if necessary, at 3–4 o'clock in the afternoon. The initial dose is usually 5 mg, two or three times daily, independent of the age or weight of the child, at 5 years of age and older. Dose–response does not vary with body weight (Rapport and Denney, 1997).

If an increase in dose is considered necessary, then increments should be small, 2.5 mg daily, at intervals not shorter than 1 week. In my experience, doses larger than 10 mg, two or three times daily, are generally not helpful and are often accompanied by unwanted side effects. Rarely, a child may require 15 or 20 mg in the morning for optimal effects on learning. Generally, if small or moderate doses of MPH are ineffective, the diagnosis and choice of treatment should be reassessed and some alternative form of stimulant or change in medication should be considered.

Twice Daily Versus Three Times Daily MPH Dose Schedule

Methylphenidate administered twice daily benefits behavior and learning of ADHD children in the classroom but not in the home. A three times daily schedule of doses may facilitate completion of homework assignments and benefit parent–child relations. In lower school grades, the twice daily dose schedule may be adequate, but in higher grades with a heavier academic load, an additional MPH dose at 3 or 4 may be required, provided sleeping habits are not disturbed. Furthermore, the third dose may prevent any MPH rebound effect experienced on returning home from school.

At the University of Chicago, the efficacy and side effects of twice daily (bid) and three times daily (tid) MPH dosing schedules (mean dose, 8 mg [0.3 mg/kg]) in 25 boys with ADHD were compared in a 5-week, placebo-controlled, crossover evaluation. Three times daily dosing provided greater improvement than the bid schedule on Conners' Parent and Teacher Rating scales, and the incidence of side effects, including insomnia, was not increased (Stein et al., 1996).

At the Hospital for Sick Children, Toronto, Canada, a placebo-controlled study of 91 children receiving MPH, titrated to 0.7 mg/kg twice daily over a period of 4 months, found that symptoms of ADHD and comorbid oppositional disorder improved while at school but not on returning home. Rebound side effects observed by parents included sadness, behavioral deterioration, irritability, withdrawal lethargy, violent behavior, and mild mania (Schachar et al., 1997).

Children in the Toronto study, receiving relatively large doses of MPH twice daily, experienced frequent rebound symptoms on returning home in the afternoon, whereas a three times daily schedule and lower doses of MPH in the Chicago study were associated with sustained improvement in behavior rating scales and much fewer side effects. Furthermore, an evening free from parent–child conflict and a homework assignment satisfactorily completed, as a result of a third dose of MPH, can lead to improved self-esteem and better classroom performance.

Safety and Effectiveness of Methylphenidate in Preschool Children with ADHD

The majority of studies of methylphenidate in ADHD have been conducted in children of 5 years and older. Parents of preschool ADHD children are often advised to rely on behavior modification counseling, a method of management that is rarely effective alone. Physicians are reluctant to prescribe stimulants for younger children because of FDA restrictions and paucity of scientifically controlled studies in children less than 6 years of age. That MPH in conservative doses may benefit learning and behavior in preschool children is demonstrated in the following study.

At the *University of Ottawa, Canada,* 31 children, aged 4–6 years, with ADHD and comorbid oppositional disorder, were treated with MPH (0.3 and 0.5 mg/kg twice daily) in a double-blind, placebo-controlled investigation. During treatment with MPH, significant improvements were obtained on a cognitive measure (number of correct responses on the Gordon Vigilance Task), on parent ratings of child's behavior, and tasks measuring the ability to complete a paper-and-pencil assignment. Improved performance during MPH treatment was also noted on measures of impulsivity-hyperactivity and conduct. Side effects, stomachache, headache, anxiety, and sadness, increased in frequency and severity with the higher dose of MPH (Musten et al., 1997).

MPH Effectiveness in ADHD Adolescents

The symptoms of ADHD in adolescents are almost identical to those during childhood, and the effectiveness and side effects of methylphenidate (MPH) are also similar in the two age groups. The dose of MPH should not automatically be increased in accordance with age and weight gains. ADHD patients who develop worsening of symptoms in high school should receive psychosocial counseling and/or tutoring before advising an increase in the dose of stimulant.

At the *Western Psychiatric Institute, University of Pittsburgh, PA,* the effectiveness of MPH, 0.3 mg/kg, in ADHD was compared during childhood and adolescence in a retrospective follow-up study of 16 patients enrolled in summer treatment programs. Of 12 objective measures of academic performance and social behavior and counselor and teacher ratings, only 3 showed significant changes in MPH responsiveness from childhood to adolescence (Smith et al., 1998).

Stimulant medication is equally effective for ADHD during childhood and adolescence, provided the environment and activities remain constant. If substance abuse becomes a problem in adolescence, it is independent of ADHD (Biederman et al., 1998). Treatment with bupropion, which has a lower abuse potential, is substituted for stimulant medication in some centers (Riggs, 1998). If substance abuse is suspected, the tamper proof, longer acting OROS formulation of methylphenidate (Concerta®) or the nonstimulant, atomoxetine (Strattera®), is the other alternative medication.

Child's Perspective of Stimulant Medication and Its Effect on Peer Relations

In a study of 45 children receiving stimulant medication for ADHD, researchers at the Boston Children's Hospital found that 89% had a favorable opinion of the treatment. Improved concentration and ability to sit still in the classroom were the most frequently reported benefits. Decreased appetite and difficulty falling asleep were the most common side effects. Only five (11%) children would prefer to discontinue medication, mainly because of the inconvenience of the lunchtime dose at school. Those taking a sustained release or long-acting stimulant found the treatment acceptable (Bowen et al., 1991).

ADHD children frequently have problems in social relationships with their peers. They are more aggressive, domineering, intrusive, and talkative, and they lack ability to communicate with others socially. Their inner or internal "locus of control" of behavior is defective, and they have a more external locus of behavior control than normal children. They view the failure to relate to others as outside their personal control and due to external factors. ADHD children, especially those with aggressive tendencies, are often rejected by their peers (Barkley, 1990; Millichap, 1998).

The effects of methylphenidate (MPH) on social behavior and peer interactions have been investigated in several studies, notably those of Carol Whalen, Barbara Henker, and colleagues at the University of California, Irvine and Los Angeles. During unstructured activities in an outside summer program, 15 of 24 hyperactive children, aged 6–11 years, treated with MPH (0.3 and 0.6 mg/kg), showed medication-related reduction in negative behavior. Younger children benefited more than older children, and the effects were dose related, using low and moderate amounts. MPH in conservative doses benefits behavior and social interaction with peers without causing social withdrawal (Whalen et al., 1987).

Treatment with stimulant medications increases compliance with parental and teacher requests and improves peer acceptance and social interaction. The reduction in aggressive behavior associated with a positive medication effect is an important factor in the improved sociability with peers (Whalen et al., 1989; Barkley, 1990).

Duration of Action of Immediate-Release and Extended-Release Formulations of Stimulant Medications for ADHD

In the past decade, several formulations of stimulant medication have been developed, each with slightly different times to onset, peak effect, and duration of action. Tables 9.1 and 9.2 show an approximation of these times for each methylphenidate and amphetamine formulation.

Immediate-Release MPH Formulations

Ritalin® and Methylin® are immediate-release, short-acting formulations of methylphenidate that act quickly and reach peak serum concentrations in 1–2 h. Their duration of effect is 3–4 h and relatively short. Doses have to be administered every 3.5–4 h during the daytime to maintain an effect. Any side effect is also short-lived, an advantage that offsets the inconvenience of multiple doses, especially during the initiation of therapy. Ritalin can be given when needed, as an aid to education, and treatment may be skipped at weekends and on vacations. Ritalin is a tablet that must be swallowed and not chewed, posing a problem for some younger children. Methylin is available as a chewable tablet or a solution for ease of administration. A rebound effect, manifested by exacerbations of hyperactivity and irritability and resulting from the rapid excretion of medication, may be troublesome on returning home from school. The rebound is prevented by the administration of a small extra dose of methylphenidate (2.5 mg) at 3 pm or by substituting an extended release formulation.

An immediate beneficial effect of a single 10 mg dose of methylphenidate on cognitive attention was demonstrated in 15 children (mean age 9 years 5 months) with ADHD compared to untreated controls (Hood et al., 2005). Cognitive improvement following a single dose of methylphenidate is predictive of improvement after 4 weeks of treatment (Buitelaar et al., 1995). High IQ, young age, and low rates of comorbid anxiety were additional predictors of a long-term response.

Focalin®, dexmethylphenidate, contains only the active D-isomer whereas Ritalin, DL-methylphenidate, is a combination of the active and inactive, L-isomer. The L-isomer is rapidly metabolized following oral ingestion and has little pharmacological effect. The dose of Focalin is one half that of methylphenidate preparations since it contains higher concentrations of the clinically active isomer. Like other immediate-release preparations, the onset of action of Focalin is fast and the peak serum concentrations are attained at 1–2 h. The duration of action is estimated at 3–6 h, and repeated daily doses should be spaced at least 4 h apart. The side effects of immediate-release Focalin are similar to those encountered with Ritalin.

Intermediate-Release MPH Formulations

Ritalin SR 20® (D,L-methylphenidate sustained release) is designed to be longer acting, approximately 7–8 h, but absorption is variable and sometimes erratic, depending on the individual. Rapid and high blood concentrations may result if the tablet is chewed rather than swallowed. Studies have found the sustained release preparation to have a delayed onset of action and to be less effective than the standard tablet, especially in the first 1 or 2 h after ingestion. It may be tried in a child who experiences behavioral rebound with the regular tablet, or in situations where in-school administration of medication is impractical or undesirable. Adults sometimes prefer Ritalin SR because it may have a lesser tendency to induce anxiety and restlessness than immediate-release Ritalin.

Methylin ER and *Metadate ER* have similar absorption characteristics to Ritalin SR. All three are intermediate-acting formulations of methylphenidate with a peak effect at 4–5 h and duration of action of 7–8 h.

Extended-Release MPH Formulations

The duration of effect of sustained- and extended-release preparations as published varies from 7–8 to 10–12 h, but individual variations occur in practice. Formulations with the longest action may be suitable for adolescents with after-school homework while the shorter acting, once a day preparations, are more appropriate for younger children. Insomnia is a more frequent side effect of some extended-release formulations. Preparations with a biphasic action may offer some advantages when addressing morning and afternoon classroom schedules. If one preparation is found ineffective, alternative stimulant formulations should be considered.

Concerta^{TM} (OROS methylphenidate HCl) is an osmotic-release oral system, extended-release formulation of methylphenidate, effective for up to 12 h after a single morning dose. Like other extended-release methylphenidate preparations, Concerta has biphasic peak activities at 1–2 and 6–8 h after oral administration. Concerta is of particular value in older child and adolescent who wish to avoid school involvement with lunchtime dosages and who require medication for completion of after-school homework or improved safety while driving an automobile.

In a controlled study of 177 adolescents with ADHD at the *Massachusetts General Hospital, Boston,* and other centers, significant improvement in symptoms was obtained in 52% of patients treated with Concerta, compared to 31% of those receiving placebo. The effects of once daily doses of 18, 36, 54, or 72 mg were compared and were significant only with the maximum dose of 72 mg. Drug-related adverse events included insomnia in 4.6%, headache in 3.4%, decreased appetite (2.3%), and diarrhea (2.3%) (Wilens et al., 2006). Improvement of the driving performance of adolescent drivers with ADHD while taking Concerta 72 mg compared to placebo was demonstrated on a driving simulator, in a study at University of Virginia, Charlottesville. The best performance occurred at 11 pm, 15 h after taking the dose of medication (Cox et al., 2006).

Focalin XR$^®$ is a once a day, extended-release formulation of dexmethylphenidate with a biphasic action and peak effects occurring at 1.5 and 6.5 h after administration. The duration of action is approximately 10–12 h. Side effects are similar to those reported for other extended-release stimulant medications.

Focalin cf Placebo. In a multicenter, controlled trial of dexmethylphenidate (D-MPH-ER) in 97 children (aged 6–17 years), a final optimal dose (mean 24 mg/day) was maintained during the last 2 weeks of the 7-week trial. Conners Scale Teacher version score improved significantly compared with placebo, and 67% patients were much improved on a Clinical Global Impressions Scale compared to 13% who received placebo. Decreased appetite, headache, and insomnia were the most common adverse events, but no patient discontinued treatment because of side effects (Greenhill et al., 2006). The mean dose of Focalin found effective (24 mg/day) is equivalent to a 50 mg/day dose of Ritalin.

Focalin XR$^®$ cf Concerta$^®$. A multicenter, double-blind, crossover study of extended release dexmethylphenidate (D-MPH-ER; Focalin XR), 20 and 30 mg/day, and D,L-methylphenidate (D,L-MPH-ER; Concerta$^®$), 36 and 54 mg/day, in 82 children, 6–12 years of age, found both drugs to be effective in treating ADHD when compared to placebo and assessed over a 12 h laboratory classroom day. D-MPH-ER had an onset of effect at 0.5 h post-dose and the duration of action was at least 12 h. D,L-MPH-ER (36 and 54 mg/day) had a slower onset of effect than D-MPH-ER (20 and 30 mg/day), but a stronger effect during the later part of the day on attention, deportment, and math test results. Both treatments were well tolerated.

The majority of adverse events were mild to moderate in severity and the most frequent were abdominal pain, decreased appetite, and headache, in more than 5% of patients (Silva et al., 2008).

Metadate CD® is an extended release preparation of methylphenidate with a biphasic action; 30% of the capsule is released rapidly, with peak effect at 1–2 h, and 70% more slowly, maximal at 4–5 h. The duration of action is 10–12 h.

Daytrana® patch contains methylphenidate in doses ranging from 10 to 30 mg. The patch is applied to the hip and is removed after 9 h. The onset of effect is delayed for 1–2 h and the duration of effect extends for 1–2 h after the patch is removed. The mean peak concentrations of D-MPH were approximately two times higher than those observed following an equal dose administered orally. The plasma concentrations varied inversely by age.

Amphetamine and Other Stimulants

Dexedrine® (dextroamphtamine), a short-acting tablet or elixir, may have a slightly longer duration of action and a slightly delayed onset compared to Ritalin.

Dexedrine Spansule® (dextroamphetamine) has a longer duration of action than the tablet form. It usually lasts for up to 12 h, with a peak effect at 7–8 h.

Adderall® (d- and D,L-amphetamines), an intermediate-release preparation, contains sulfate, aspartate, and saccharate salts that provide a steadier level of amphetamines for up to 5–7 h. It has a longer duration of action than Ritalin (Swanson et al., 1998), and a single morning dose may suffice. The effect on attention and behavior is smoother and more sustained than methylphenidate, with lesser tendency toward withdrawal irritability and rebound side effects. It is supplied in capsule form as sprinkles, permitting easier administration with food, if required in small children who are unable to swallow pills.

Adderall XR®, an extended-release form, reaches a peak level at 7–8 h and the effect may last for 12 h. In a long-term 24-month, multicenter, open-label, placebo-controlled trial of Adderall XR in 568 children, aged 6–12 years, significant improvements (>30%) in a Conners Global Index Scale, Parents version, were maintained. Adverse events included anorexia (15%), headache (15%), and insomnia (11%); 15% withdrew from the study because of adverse events. Serious adverse events occurred in 3%, including convulsions in two patients, at doses 10 and 20 mg/day. Mean systolic blood pressure increased by 3.5 mmHg, diastolic by 2.6 mmHg, and pulse rate by 3.4 beats per min (McGough et al., 2005).

Vyvanse® (lisdexamfetamine dimesylate) is a relatively new amphetamine pro-drug introduced as an extended release treatment for ADHD. Several clinical trials have demonstrated short- (4 weeks) and long-term (11 months) effectiveness and a tolerability profile similar to those of other extended-release stimulants (Biederman et al., 2007; Lopez et al., 2008; Findling et al., 2008).

Cylert® (pemoline) is a long-acting stimulant that was popular in the 1970s as an alternative to Ritalin, when a single daily dose was preferred. After reports of liver toxicity, Cylert was no longer recommended in 1995 and is now unavailable in the United States (Hochman et al., 1998; Shevell and Schreiber, 1997; Rosh et al., 1998).

Provigil® (modafinil) is a novel wakefulness promoting agent, approved for treatment of narcolepsy in adults and adolescents over 16 years. The mechanism of action of modafinil is related to an increase in dopamine levels and blocked dopamine transporters in the brain (Volkow et al., 2009). Trials in children with ADHD have shown significant improvements in attentiveness. Adverse effects include insomnia (29%), headache (20%), and decreased appetite (16%). Serious side effects prompting drug withdrawal in 3% included erythema multiforme, Stevens–Johnson syndrome, somnolence, dystonia, and tachycardia (Biederman et al., 2005). Modafinil adverse reactions and potential for abuse are a concern in this choice of alternative medication for ADHD.

Duration of Treatment with Stimulant Medication

Parents are frequently concerned that treatment with stimulants has to be continued indefinitely. In practice, the average child will receive treatment intermittently for 3 years. Some will be able to discontinue medication after 1 year and others may need therapy for 5 years or longer (Millichap, 1996; Millichap, 1997).

Duration of stimulant therapy is determined by trial and error. Drug holidays during extended summer vacations permit reappraisal of the need for medication on return to school. Teacher reports regarding attention and behavior should be obtained within 1–2 weeks after starting a new term. In children whose symptoms of ADHD are persistent, the physician should be consulted about renewal of a prescription.

Researchers find little evidence of abuse or overuse of stimulant medication during treatment of ADHD in childhood and adolescence (Goldman et al., 1998). Based on DEA production quotas for methylphenidate (MPH), a 2.8-fold increase in usage between 1990 and 1995 is far less than the media claims of a 6-fold increased usage. Approximately 2.8% (1.5 million) US children aged 5–18 received MPH for ADHD in 1995. The increased usage was related to more prolonged treatment, more girls treated, and adolescents receiving medication for ADD (Safer et al., 1996).

Long-Term Usage of Stimulants and Outcome of ADHD

Studies of long-term, uninterrupted stimulant therapy for ADHD are infrequent. One recent report of a 15-month controlled trial of amphetamine in 62 children, aged 6–11 years, showed continued improvements in behavior and learning ability, with no serious side effects. A multicenter, placebo-controlled trial of amphetamine treatment for ADHD in Sweden found significant improvements in attention, hyperactivity, and disruptive behaviors and a mean change in IQ of +4.5 after more than 9 months of amphetamine sulfate. Side effects included decreased appetite in 56%, abdominal pain in 32%, tics in 29%, and visual hallucinations requiring dose reduction or withdrawal in 5%. Abdominal pain and tics occurred with equal frequency in the placebo group, and only one of 4 children with tics at baseline had an increase in symptoms during amphetamine (15 mg/day) treatment (Gillberg et al., 1997).

The children in the Swedish study had a high incidence of comorbid diagnoses (42%), including pervasive developmental disorders, mild retardation, and oppositional defiant disorder. Long-term trials of stimulants in ADHD with less comorbidity would be expected to show greater beneficial effects and a lower incidence of side effects. The unusually high incidence of tic disorders in both treated and untreated children was remarkable.

Continuity of Therapy with Immediate-Release cf Extended-Release Methylphenidate

Compared to immediate-release MPH-treated children (aged 6–17 years), patients treated with extended-release MPH had a significantly longer mean duration of sustained treatment (140 vs 103 days, respectively). Comparing ER-MPH formulations, Concerta treatment was continued longer than Metadate CD or Ritalin SR (147, 113, and 101 days, respectively) (Marcus et al., 2005). Overall, less than one half of the patients continued therapy beyond 90 days, and less than 20% continued for 1 year. Long-acting formulations prolong compliance and continuity of therapy; treatment with Concerta having a 12-h duration of action is maintained longer than Ritalin LA, which is effective for only 8 h.

Multimodal Treatment Study of ADHD (MTA)

A collaborative multimodal treatment study of children with ADHD, the MTA (Jensen et al., 1997), was organized by the National Institute of Mental Health (NIMH) and collaborators to compare long-term effectiveness of various treatment strategies. Patients were assigned to one of the following four groups: (1) medication alone, (2) combined medication/behavior modification, (3) behavior modification alone, and (4) routine community care. The first patients were enrolled in 1994 and the study was completed in 1998. A total of 579 children were enrolled in the study, and 540 (93%) participated in the first follow-up at 10 months after the 14 months of intensive intervention. At both the initial follow-up and reassessment at 24 months, the MTA medication strategy showed persisting significant superiority over behavior modification and community care for ADHD and ODD, but the benefits of medication at 24 months had diminished as compared to the outcome at 10 months. Combination medication and behavior therapy was not superior to medical management alone, and the results of behavior therapy were not significantly different from community care. The benefits of intensive medical management for

ADHD symptoms extend 10 months beyond the treatment phase but the effects diminish over time (NIMH, 2004).

A 2005 overview and analysis of current literature on the treatment of ADHD by the American Academy of Pediatrics Committee on Quality Improvement concluded the following: (1) ADHD should be managed as a chronic condition; (2) stimulant medications are beneficial and different stimulants are equally effective; (3) behavioral therapy is minimally effective but only in combination with medication; and (4) education and counseling of patient and family are necessary adjuncts to drug therapy (Brown et al. Pediatrics 2005).

Prolonged Usage of MPH Through Adolescence and Young Adulthood and Risks of Motor Vehicle Accidents Related to ADHD

ADHD young adults are twice as likely to be cited for unlawful speeding and have more crashes and more accidents involving bodily injury, when compared to non-ADHD adult control subjects. They are more likely to have licenses suspended, and their driving habits and performance are poorer despite adequate driving knowledge. These statistics were obtained from a study of motor vehicle skills, risks, and accidents in 25 young adults with ADHD compared to controls, aged 17–30 years, followed at the University of Massachusetts Medical Center, Worcester, MA (Barkley et al., 1996).

This study confirms previous reports of an increased incidence of motor vehicle accidents and injury among ADHD young adults. The findings support a proposed need for continued treatment and supervision of adolescents with ADHD into adulthood, particularly in patients with persistent problems in motor control and impulsive behavior (Mannuzza et al., 1998).

Side Effects of Stimulant Medications

Side Effects of Methylphenidate and Their Prevalence

Side effects of methylphenidate (MPH) are generally mild and transient. Prolonged medical usage of MPH for more than 40 years has failed to uncover any life-threatening toxic reactions. The list and frequency of occurrence of the most common side effects of MPH are shown in Table 9.3. They are usually dose related. These data are based on personal experience as well as reviews of the medical literature (Barkley et al., 1991; Ahmann et al., 1993). The significance of reported MPH-related side effects is assessed by comparison with symptoms occurring during drug "holidays," at weekends and on vacations, and by placebo-controlled trials.

Table 9.3 Side effects of methylphenidate

Side effect	Dose-related occurrence (%)	
	Low dose	Moderate dose
Decreased appetite	40	60
Increased appetite	5	5
Insomnia	10	15
Stomachaches	10	15
Weight loss	5	10
Headaches	3	5
Tics	3	5
Mood change	2	7
Growth delay	1	5

Decreased appetite occurs in about 50% of patients taking MPH. The child eats lunch sparingly but often has a good appetite for dinner. If weight loss occurs, it usually stabilizes after 4 weeks, provided the dosage of MPH is small to moderate. Dietary supplements (Pediasure, Ensure) offered at breakfast and bedtime are usually sufficient to compensate for the reduced appetite at lunchtime. Appetite stimulation may occur in a small percentage of patients; ironically, this occurs usually in those who are overweight before starting the treatment.

Insomnia occurs mainly when MPH is taken after 4 o'clock in the afternoon or when higher or extended-release doses are required. A modification of the timing or size of dose permits a return to normal sleep habits.

Stomachaches and headaches are sometimes troublesome, necessitating either reduction in dosage or a change in diet. Headaches due to tension and school frustrations are often relieved when MPH is begun.

Tics, mood changes, and growth delay are side effects that may cause greater concern, and these are discussed in more detail.

Effect of Medication on Growth of Children with ADHD

A suppressant effect of stimulant drugs on the growth of hyperactive children was reported in 1972 (Safer D et al.). The annual growth lag was minimal (1.0–1.5 cm) and occurred only when larger doses (>20 mg daily) of methylphenidate (MPH) or dextroamphetamine were given regularly for 2 or more years. An analysis of heights of 50 children in my practice failed to confirm a growth suppressant effect of MPH, when more conservative doses were used and treatment was interrupted at weekends and on vacations (Millichap, 1977).

Growth delays caused by MPH are a major concern of parents partly because of excess media attention to this side effect. In reality, growth is delayed only with higher doses and when weight loss is significant. A rebound in growth to normal levels may be expected when treatment is interrupted, and permanent growth suppression does not occur. Indeed, a stimulation of growth has been observed in some younger patients.

A review in 2005 found 29 reports of studies of growth, 22 in children and 7 in late adolescents, in relation to stimulant medication for ADHD. Of 21 reports classified by study design, 9 showed statistically significant attenuation of growth in height and 12 showed normal growth patterns. The average height deficit estimated during the first 1–3 years of treatment was approximately 1 cm/year. No or lesser attenuation occurred in patients taking methylphenidate in doses not exceeding 20 mg/day. More attenuation of growth occurred with dextroamphetamine treatment and in patients with gastrointestinal side effects. Initial weight loss precedes the effect on growth, and increments in height take time to adjust to a new equilibrium during stimulant therapy. With rare exceptions, children achieve a satisfactory adult height. A rebound in growth generally occurs during the third year of treatment or after medication is discontinued. In two studies, the weight centile stabilized while the height centile continued to decline for the third and fourth year. Of the six studies of late adolescents or patients followed to adulthood with ADHD, none showed any significant difference in growth between those treated with stimulants during childhood and the controls (Poulton, 2005).

The NIMH Multimodal Treatment Study found the group of patients treated consistently for 14 months with medication showed reduced growth rate at 24-month follow-up, compared to the group on no medication. Significant growth suppression had occurred in the combination and medical management groups after 14 months of the treatment phase (NIMD/MTA Cooperative Group, 2004). Consistent treatment reduced the rate of growth but lengthened the duration of growth. Adult height would be delayed but not reduced. The hypothesis that an initial growth suppression will be followed by a growth rebound, even when medication is continued through summer vacation (Satterfield et al., 1979), is not supported by the MTA study.

Despite the evidence for a stimulant-induced retardation in growth, many studies show no adverse effect on growth. In fact, a possible growth stimulant effect was noted with modest doses of methylphenidate in 6 of 36 patients less than 8 years of age (Millichap, 1977). Discrepancies in findings between studies may depend on several factors, the most important related to dose of stimulant and the use of drug holidays, weekends, and vacations. Studies employing smaller doses of 20 mg/day or less and on school days only are generally free from adverse effects on growth. The use of extended-release stimulant medications may also introduce a further reason for careful monitoring of height and weight.

The effect of OROS methylphenidate (Concerta®) (34–43 mg daily) on the height and weight of 178 children, aged 6–13 years, treated for at least 21 months for ADHD, was evaluated at the *Massachusetts General Hospital, Boston* (Spencer et al., 2006). Their height steadily increased throughout the study and weight showed no change, but on average patients' height was 0.23 cm less and weight 1.23 kg less than expected at 21 months. Those taking drug holidays showed lesser decreases in weight and growth. The authors conclude that the effects of Concerta on growth are clinically insignificant, and decreases in weight are limited to the first month of therapy.

Obesity in Children Untreated for ADHD

Of all the ADHD children studied at *Brown Medical School, Providence, RI*, 21% were overweight, 15.5% were at the risk of being overweight, 6.7% were under-weight, and 56.7% were of normal weight. Patients not treated with medication had −1.5 times the odds of being overweight whereas those currently medicated had − 1.6 times the odds of being underweight, as compared to controls without ADHD. The weight status in ADHD children was independent of gender, race, ethnicity, socioeconomic status, or depression or anxiety. Behavior patterns might explain the increased risk of obesity (Waring and Lapane 2008).

Mood Changes Sometimes Associated with MPH and Their Avoidance

Irritability, a tendency to cry easily, impassive expression, and dysphoria or sadness are some of the mood changes reported in children taking methylphenidate (MPH) and other stimulant medications. "My child looks like a zombi," is a parent's usual response to this side effect. Depressive reactions to MPH occur mainly with larger doses (20 mg, 2 or 3× daily or higher) and in children with a family history of depression. Irritability may also occur as a "rebound" phenomenon, on returning home from school in the afternoon. A small dose of MPH (5 mg) given at 3 pm or a reduction in the lunchtime dose will usually correct this withdrawal effect.

The dose-related dysphoric (depressive) effect of MPH and other stimulants is usually accompanied by a loss of appetite and weight. It can be avoided by either reduction in dosage or a change to an alternative medication.

Management of Tics Developing During Stimulant Therapy for ADHD

Tics or Tourette syndrome may develop as a side effect of stimulant therapy for ADHD, especially in children with a prior history or family predisposition to tic disorders. Rarely, obsessive compulsive disorder is also associated with tics and MPH therapy. The frequency of occurrence of transient tics is approximately 5%, or 1 in 20 patients treated. Some have estimated that fewer than 1% of ADHD children treated with methylphenidate will develop a tic disorder, whereas the risk is closer to 10% in patients with a pre-existing tendency to tics (Denckla et al., 1976).

Parents should be alert to the symptoms of tics or Tourette syndrome, and the physician should be notified if tics develop. Stimulants of all types, includ-ing caffeine-containing beverages and chocolate, should generally be avoided in patients with a tendency to tics. Withdrawal of the stimulant is usually followed by remission but rarely, tics may persist and require therapy. MPH appears less likely to induce persistent tic exacerbations than amphetamines.

   At the National Institute of Mental Health, Bethesda, MD, the effects of methylphenidate (MPH) and dextroamphetamine (DEX) on tic severity in 20 boys with ADHD and comorbid Tourette syndrome were investigated in a 9-week, placebo-controlled, double-blind crossover study. Tic severity was significantly greater during treatment with high doses of both MPH (20–25 mg twice daily) and DEX (12.5–22.5 mg twice daily). ADHD symptoms were benefited by both stimulants, and treatment was continued for 1–3 years in 14 of the 20 patients. Tic exacerbations were reversible and MPH was better tolerated than DEX (Castellanos et al., 1997). Conventional doses of MPH (0.1–0.3 mg/kg) produced dramatic improvement in behavior in children with ADHD and tic disorders, in a study *at State University of New York, Stony Brook, NY* (Nolan and Gadow, 1997).

   The occurrence of tics with MPH or amphetamines is generally dose related, occurring mainly with larger doses. The lowest effective dose of stimulant should be used, and increases in dosage should be made slowly. If a reduction in dose is not quickly followed by a remission of tics, then the stimulant should be discontinued.

   Clonidine (Catapres®) is an alternative medication prescribed in children with ADHD complicated by tics. Combinations of clonidine and stimulant drugs are usually not advised, since serious cardiac-related adverse effects are occasionally reported. Physicians differ in practice; personally, I withdraw the stimulant before introducing clonidine (See Chap. 7 and a subsequent section on use of clonidine for tics).

Behavioral Rebound Associated with MPH Treatment for ADHD

Some children with ADHD treated with morning and noon doses of methylphenidate (MPH) will function satisfactorily at school, but their behavior relapses when they return home in the afternoon. This deterioration in behavior, sometimes exceeding the pre-treatment condition, is called "behavioral rebound." It is characterized by an increase in hyperactivity and impulsiveness and, in addition, the child becomes irritable, tends to cry easily, and may have temper outbursts. In a sample of 21 children treated with two doses of MPH, about one third were affected by behavioral deterioration in late afternoon or evening, and the degree of rebound was variable from day to day (Johnston et al., 1988).

   Treatment options for behavioral rebound include the addition of a small dose (2.5 or 5 mg) of MPH at 3 or 4 o'clock in the afternoon, or a reduction in the noontime dosage. Alternatively, a change to a longer acting stimulant such as Ritalin SR or Adderall may be found satisfactory.

Methylphenidate and Exacerbation of Seizures

The relation of seizures to treatment with methylphenidate (MPH) is controversial. A tendency to seizures demonstrated by an abnormal electroencephalogram occurs in 7% or more of children with ADHD, and clinical seizures are occasionally reported in children taking larger doses of MPH and other stimulants (Millichap and Swisher, 1997). Patients taking combinations of MPH and antidepressants, such as imipramine, bupropion, or sertraline, are especially at risk of seizures.

The Physicians' Desk Reference (PDR) includes a contraindication to the use of Ritalin® as follows: "There is some clinical evidence that Ritalin may lower the convulsive threshold in patients with prior history of seizures, with prior EEG abnormalities in the absence of seizures, and, very rarely, in absence of history of seizures and no prior EEG evidence of seizures. Safe concomitant use of anticonvulsants and Ritalin has not been established. In the presence of seizures, the drug should be discontinued."

While the PDR cautions against the use of MPH in patients with epilepsy and ADHD, most neurologists will prescribe MPH or other stimulant therapy, provided that seizures are controlled with adequate levels of antiepileptic medications. In studies of children with well-controlled epilepsy and ADHD, the addition of MPH to antiepileptic drug therapy had no adverse effect on seizure control or on the EEG. MPH can be a safe and effective treatment for ADHD complicated by epilepsy, provided that seizures are controlled by anticonvulsant medication (McBride et al., 1986; Feldman et al., 1989; Gross-Tsur et al., 1997). MPH should be discontinued or the dosage reduced, if seizures recur. Combinations of MPH and some antidepressants will increase the risk of seizures and should be avoided.

At Wright State University, School of Medicine, Dayton, OH, a 13-year-old boy with ADHD and depressive reaction had a tonic-clonic seizure 1 week after the antidepressant sertraline (50 mg/day) was added to treatment with MPH (80 mg/day). MPH dosage had been gradually increased without seizure occurrence over a period of a year before the addition of sertraline. The EEG was normal. Sertraline was discontinued, and MPH was continued unchanged with no recurrence of seizures (Feeney and Klykylo, 1997).

An EEG is indicated if a child with ADHD has a personal or family history of seizures, or recurrent staring episodes. If the EEG is epileptiform but no clinical seizures have occurred, a trial of small doses of MPH may be initiated followed by EEG monitoring at intervals. MPH may be continued in the absence of seizures or worsening of the EEG. In children with ADHD complicated by EEG centrotemporal (rolandic) spikes, 16.7% developed seizures compared to 0.6% in a group of ADHD children with normal EEGs (Hemmer et al., 2001).

Although MPH may exacerbate epileptiform activity in the EEG of patients susceptible to seizures, one study in non-seizure patients with ADHD demonstrated a normalizing effect. Using EEG spectral analysis in 23 boys with ADHD, regional improvements in the EEG during MPH treatment were associated with improvements in tasks involving reading, coding, and visual—motor perception. The EEG as a measure of MPH effects in ADHD requires further study (Swartwood et al., 1998).

The choice of antiepileptic medication in children with ADHD and seizures is important. Certain drugs, particularly phenobarbital, will exacerbate hyperactivity, and many of the antiepileptic medications can affect learning and memory at therapeutic dose levels.

Unusual Side Effects of Methylphenidate and Other Stimulants

The following side effects of MPH occur infrequently but may require reduction in dosage or withdrawal of the drug and substitution of an alternative therapy:

- *Increase in hyperactivity* occurs in 5% of children treated with MPH. Other forms of stimulant medications will have the same effect in these individual patients, and a different class of treatment will be indicated. The antihypertensive agent, clonidine, or the antidepressant, bupropion, is an alternative choice of drug therapy.
- *Obsessive compulsive disorder* (OCD) is a rarely reported side effect of MPH and is sometimes associated with tics. Dextroamphetamine has been implicated more often than MPH. An 8-year-old boy developed a transient but severely debilitating OCD after 2 weeks of treatment with MPH (10 mg/daily) for a mild, uncomplicated ADHD. He also developed tics involving the head and neck. The past history was negative for psychiatric comorbidity, recent streptococcal infection, and familial anxiety disorders. Withdrawal of MPH was followed by gradual recovery from OCD over a 3-month period (Kouris, 1998).
- *Trichotillomania*, a compulsive habit of hair pulling from the scalp, eyebrows, and even eyelashes, is an occasional side effect of MPH. In one study involving 3 boys, symptoms abated in 2, despite continuation of the MPH. The habit persisted in one after switching to imipramine (Martin et al., 1998). Females are affected 10 times more often than males, and depressive symptoms are common (Keuthen et al., 1998).
- *Hallucinations* (visual or tactile sensations of insects or snakes), psychosis or mania, occur in 11/743 (1.48/100) person-years in pooled data from 49 controlled studies and in >800 postmarketing reports (Mosholder et al., 2009). Of 11 cases, transdermal methylphenidate accounted for four and the nonstimulant, atomoxetine, also for four.
- *Fingertip skin and nail-biting* occurs in 1–3% of patients after starting MPH and appears to be related to the treatment. A reduction in dosage may be sufficient to correct this side effect.
- *Redness and burning sensation* in the ears, face, and hands are side effects of MPH in 1% of children.
- *Peeling of the skin* of the palms is a rare observation and a suspect but not proven side effect of MPH. A reduction in dose and sometimes withdrawal of the drug may be necessary.
- *Generalized skin rash* is a rare side effect, occurring in less than 0.5% of children. A drug-related skin rash is an indication to discontinue treatment.
- Complete blood counts and liver function tests are generally recommended at 6-month intervals or if indicated by specific symptoms. Routine testing is not generally necessary if medication is withheld at weekends and on vacations.

- *Cardiac complications.* Palpitations, rapid pulse, chest pain, and elevated blood pressure occur infrequently, particularly with larger doses of MPH. An electrocardiogram and cardiology consultation are recommended, and the stimulant medication should be discontinued or the dose reduced.
- *Immune system disorder.* A possible effect on the immune system by MPH in larger doses (30–45 mg/day) is reported in an isolated study (Auci et al., 1997). MPH induced a twofold increase in IgE levels in three out of six boys treated, as well as in other signs of immune system hypersensitivity. Larger doses of MPH should be avoided when possible, especially in patients with IgE-mediated asthma, allergic rhinitis, and other atopic diseases. Drugs used in asthma have been implicated as a cause of ADHD. If significant, this study warns of a possible adverse effect of MPH on the outcome of asthma and other allergic diseases.

Alternative Medications to Stimulants

Approximately 20–25% of children with ADHD fail to respond to stimulant medication or have side effects or conditions contraindicating their use. Table 9.4 lists the generic and brand names of alternative drugs and the strength of tablets or other forms.

Table 9.4 Alternative medications to stimulants in treatment of ADHD

Generic name	Brand name	Form	Strength (mg)
Atomoxetine	Strattera	Capsule	10, 18, 25, 40, 60
Clonidine	Catapres	Tablet	0.1
	Catapres TTS	Patch	0.1
Guanfacine	Tenex	Tablet	1.0
Bupropion	Wellbutrin	Tablet	75, 100
	Wellbutrin SR	Tablet	100, 150

Alternative medications for ADHD that may be substituted when stimulant therapy fails include the non-stimulant atomoxetine (Strattera®), antihypertensive agents, clonopin (Catapres®) or guanfacine (Tenex®), and the antidepressant, bupropion (Wellbutrin®) (Table 9.4). Other forms of antidepressants (tricyclics, imipramine, and desipramine) are offered as second-line treatments for ADHD in children under psychiatric care (Malhotra and Santosh, 1998). Anticonvulsant medications have variable effects on behavior and attention but some may benefit hyperactive children with seizure disorders.

Each of these drugs has specific indications in addition to ADHD. These include the occurrence of comorbid disorders such as tics, oppositional defiance and conduct disorders, mood disorders, and seizures. The choice of medication is dependent not only on efficacy but also on the type and prevalence of reported side effects. In treating children with ADHD, the safety of a medication and absence of serious adverse reactions are of foremost importance in the physician's selection.

Indications for the Nonstimulant, Atomoxetine (Strattera®), Usage, and Side Effects

Patients with ADHD complicated by tics, Tourette syndrome, seizures, or sleep disorders may develop worsening of these symptoms if stimulants are used. Strattera may be a first choice medication in these situations. Strattera is effective in the inattentive, hyperactive, and combined types of ADHD and is not intended as a substitute for stimulant medication only in the inattentive type. Similarly, methylphenidate and amphetamine preparations are effective in all subtypes of ADHD.

Strattera® is a selective norepinephrine reuptake inhibitor. Capsules are available in strengths as low as 10 mg and as high as 80 and 100 mg, for use in adults. The usual dosage based on body weight is 0.5 mg/kg initially, increasing to a target daily dose of 1.2 mg/kg. No additional benefit has been demonstrated for doses higher than 1.2 mg/kg. Capsules are taken orally in the morning after breakfast or in the evening after dinner. The evening dose is recommended if drowsiness is a side effect with morning doses.

Strattera® is contraindicated in patients with high blood pressure, heart disease, glaucoma, or liver dysfunction. Liver enzymes should be determined before beginning therapy. It should not be taken with monoamine oxidase inhibitor drugs (MAOIs). Adverse events most commonly reported, and that can require discontinuance in 5% or more patients, include appetite decrease, stomach upset, nausea, vomiting, fatigue, drowsiness, dizziness, and mood swings. Suicidal thoughts (but no attempts) are reported, and a black box warning is issued.

Suicidal ideation occurred in 0.4% (5/1357) children and adolescents in short-term (6–18 weeks) trials of Strattera compared to none in placebo-treated patients (851 patients). Patients should be monitored closely for suicidal thinking or behavior.

Long-Term Effects of Strattera® on Growth and Blood Pressure in Children with ADHD

A meta-analysis of seven double-blind/placebo-controlled and six open-label studies found that effectiveness of Strattera was maintained in 70% of 97 children, aged 6–7 years, treated for >2 years. Twenty-five percent discontinued therapy because of lack of effectiveness and 4% because of adverse events. Height and weight measurements after 24 months of treatment were 2.7 cm and 2.5 kg less than expected. Significant increases in pulse rate (7.2 bpm), diastolic BP (3.4 mmHg), and systolic BP (3.7 mm/kg) were noted. ECG-corrected QT interval increase of 0.2 ms was

not significant, but PR interval was significantly shortened with a mean change of
−4.3 s (*P*<0.001) (Kratochvil et al., 2006). Strattera has similar effects to stimulants
on growth, weight gain, and cardiovascular function.

A significant elevation in blood pressure was noted in three adolescent boys
while taking atomoxetine in a dose of 80 mg/day (Dworkin, 2005). An 11-year-old
boy with ADHD developed palpitations and repolarization changes in the electrocardiogram after 10 months of standard dose treatment (1.1 mg/kg/day) with
atomoxetine (Rajesh et al., 2006). The echocardiogram was normal. Symptoms and
ECG abnormalities resolved when atomoxetine was discontinued. Growth and cardiac monitoring is recommended during treatment with Strattera, similar to that
followed for stimulant medication for ADHD.

Dopamine Transporter DAT1 Genotype and Response to Atomoxetine cf Methylphenidate

A genetic variation in DAT1, a known link to risk of ADHD and a site of action
of methylphenidate, may influence the neurophysiological effects of methylphemi-
date and atomoxetine. Methylphenidate and atomoxetine had similar effects on short
interval-cortical inhibition (SICI), measured in motor cortex with transcranial magnetic stimulation, but their effects differed significantly by DAT1 genotype. Both
drugs increased SICI toward normal in heterozygotes but not in 10-repeat homozy-
gotes (Gilbert et al., 2006). ADHD patients with the DAT1 10/10 homozygous
genotype respond poorly to methylphenidate.

Indications for Clonidine or Guanfacine in ADHD

Clonidine (Catapres®) is a second-line treatment for ADHD and is indicated primarily in patients with a history or complication of tics or Tourette syndrome.
Behavioral symptoms of ADHD and tics are expected to respond, but inattentiveness
and distractibility may persist. Children with comorbid oppositional defiance disorder, anger, and low frustration tolerance may be benefited. Drowsiness and fatigue
are the most frequent side effects, but given at bedtime to a child with poor sleeping
habits, a clonidine side effect may convert to a benefit.

The initial daily dose is small, beginning with one-quarter or one-half tablet
(0.025–0.05 mg) 1 h after the evening meal or 1 h before bedtime. At least 7 days
to 2 weeks should be allowed before expecting optimal effects of clonidine on daytime behavior. If no benefit is obtained after 2 weeks, the daily dose is increased by
one-half tablet in the morning after breakfast, provided the child is not drowsy. A
further increase of one-quarter or one-half tablet in the afternoon, on return home
from school, may be made if necessary, but increments should be made slowly and
not sooner than 5–7 day intervals. The optimal dose tolerated in children, 5–14 years
of age, is usually 0.1–0.15 mg daily, but larger amounts are sometimes required.

When clonidine is first prescribed, parents and teachers are advised to be patient while judging the response. Unlike methylphenidate that acts within hours, the beneficial effects of clonidine on ADHD may be delayed for days or weeks.

Clonidine treatment should not be interrupted at weekends. Sudden withdrawal of larger doses may cause blood pressure elevation or "rebound," hyperactivity, headache, agitation, or exacerbated tics. If treatment is omitted during long vacations, withdrawal should be made slowly and tapered over 4–7 days.

Adverse Effects of Clonidine

In addition to drowsiness, occasionally serious and sometimes fatal, reactions to clonidine are reported when taken in combination with methylphenidate or other stimulant. Four cases of adverse reactions to clonidine, administered in combination with MPH or Dexedrine, in children aged 8–10 years, are reported from the *University of California, LA* (Cantwell et al., 1997). One patient taking clonidine 0.1 mg 3x daily and MPH 20 mg 2x daily became sedated and fatigued, the blood pressure and pulse were 30% below baseline readings, an electrocardiogram showed slowing and irregular heart rhythms, and the Holter heart monitor recorded an irregular and slow heart rate in sleep.

A second patient, while on clonidine 0.1 mg in the evening and Dexedrine 12.5 mg daily, forgot to take one clonidine dose. After rollerblading for 10 min, she became tremulous, her breathing and swallowing were impaired, she looked terrified, her respiration and pulse were abnormally rapid, she became combative, hallucinated, and disorientated and febrile. The next morning she had recovered and had no memory for the event.

A third patient, prescribed clonidine 0.15 mg in the evening, methylphenidate 50 mg/daily, and lithium, had a slow pulse and an abnormal electrocardiogram with signs of heart block. The fourth patient had recurrent episodes of fainting related to exercise during treatment with a clonidine patch, 0.2 mg every 5 days. He complained of faintness, passed out, convulsed, and died of cardiac arrest after swimming for 45 min. An autopsy revealed a previously undiagnosed congenital heart malformation with stenosis of the left coronary artery. Clonidine blood levels were normal.

Guidelines for Use of Clonidine in Treating ADHD

The following guidelines for use of clonidine in the treatment of ADHD are recommended:

- Combination therapy with MPH, other stimulants, or antidepressants should be avoided when possible or used with caution (Daviss et al., 2008);
- Screen for history of heart disease, and examine heart sounds, pulse, and blood pressure. Obtain EKG and cardiac consultation for abnormal readings, murmurs, or exercise-related syncopal symptoms;

- Dose changes should not exceed 0.05 mg every 5–7 days;
- Parents should be aware that the safety and effectiveness of clonidine and Catapres-TTS® have not been endorsed by the FDA for use in children;
- Children who have taken clonidine for more than a few weeks should not stop the drug abruptly. Withdrawal symptoms, including increased blood pressure, anxiety, and agitation, may result.

Guanfacine (Tenex®) is an antihypertensive agent with action and side effects similar to clonidine. Guanfacine may have a slightly less sedative effect than clonidine and a longer duration of action.

Bupropion (Wellbutrin®) is a novel antidepressant, chemically unrelated to other agents, which blocks the uptake by neurons of the neurotransmitters, serotonin, and norepinephrine. Although generally indicated for use in adults, the effectiveness of Wellbutrin in the treatment of ADHD in children has been demonstrated in several controlled studies (Simeon et al., 1986; Casat et al., 1987; Clay et al., 1988). Wellbutrin is usually well tolerated and is a useful alternative, when first-line stimulant medications are ineffective or associated with serious side effects. It may also be indicated in patients with ADHD complicated by mood disorders. In one controlled study, comparing treatment with bupropion and methylphenidate in 15 children with ADHD, both drugs were effective, rating scales tending to favor MPH (Barrickman et al., 1995).

Bupropion has a slightly higher risk of causing or exacerbating seizures than other antidepressants, especially in patients with a history of eating disorders. It should not be prescribed with other drugs known to lower the seizure threshold. Bupropion is not recommended in patients with a personal or family history of epilepsy or an abnormal EEG, unless seizures are controlled by antiepileptic medications.

Side effects of bupropion, also seen with methylphenidate and amphetamines, include an exacerbation of tics in children with comorbid ADHD and Tourette syndrome (Spencer et al., 1993), and the occurrence of insomnia at the beginning of treatment. Tics and Tourette syndrome may be a contraindication to its use. Insomnia may be prevented by avoiding bedtime doses. Other occasional side effects in children include skin rash, swollen lips, nausea, increased appetite, tremor, and agitation (Casat, 1987; Clay, 1988; Dulcan, 1994).

Carbamazepine (Tegretol®) is an anticonvulsant, especially effective in complex partial and generalized tonic-clonic seizures. It also has some mood-stabilizing properties. Several studies reporting the results of carbamazepine (CBZ) therapy for ADHD show that 70% of patients are improved. Hyperactivity, impulsivity, and distractibility were controlled following treatment with CBZ, and the longer the treatment the better the outcome.

In 3 placebo-controlled, double-blind studies, 71% of 53 patients treated with CBZ were benefited whereas only 26% of 52 receiving placebo showed improvements in attentiveness and behavior. The difference was significant. Side effects, mainly drowsiness and skin rash, were reported in 7% of patients (Silva et al., 1996).

CBZ may be a useful alternative therapy for ADHD, especially in patients with a history of epilepsy or with an abnormal electroencephalogram (EEG). A review of the literature revealed that 70–80% of the patients with ADHD benefited by treatment with CBZ had abnormal EEGs (Millichap, 1997a). Most antiepileptic medications, including CBZ, may cause cognitive impairment and impulsivity in patients treated for epilepsy. Treatment with CBZ must be monitored with measurements of drug levels, blood counts, and liver function tests.

Carbatrol®, a carbamazepine extended-release capsule, recently introduced, may be swallowed whole, or the contents sprinkled on food, for ease of administration. Like Tegretol-XR tablet form, Carbatrol is taken twice daily.

Trileptal®, oxcarbazepine, is an alternative anticonvulsant to Tegretol, with similar effectiveness and lesser incidence of side effects.

Depakote®, valproate. Extended-release valproate was effective in the treatment of three boys with ADHD-hyperactive-impulsive type associated with giant somatosensory-evoked potentials (SEP). SEP amplitudes following median nerve stimulation were decreased to normal voltage in 2 patients after treatment with valproate (Miyazaki et al., 2006). The authors recommend testing SEP in methylphenidate nonresponders and valproate considered in patients with giant SEP.

Well-Tried Stimulant Medications Versus Novel Less-Established Remedies for ADHD

A number of alternative and less well-tried medications are sometimes prescribed for the treatment of ADHD. Ritalin® (methylphenidate) is the mainstay of the drug therapies available, its effectiveness and safety having been established for more than 40 years. Other stimulants, Dexedrine® and Adderall®, are also effective and are sometimes substituted, according to the preference of the physician. Strattera® is prescribed in preference to stimulants in patients with tics, seizures, or insomnia. Antihypertensive agents, Catapres® (clonidine) and Tenex® (guanfacine), are indicated in children with ADHD complicated by tics or comorbid oppositional defiance and aggression, and the antidepressant agent, Wellbutrin® (bupropion), is of value in children with ADHD and comorbid mood disorders or those failing to respond to stimulants. The tricyclic antidepressants are sometimes prescribed as second-line therapy for ADHD. However, the cardiovascular side effects, rarely resulting in fatalities, are a major concern, and careful monitoring and caution are essential (Wilens et al., 1996).

Novel medications with promise include Focalin®, a congener of methylphenidate, and Vyvanse®, an amphetamine. Early trials of both of these agents have demonstrated effectiveness and advantages compared to conventional medications. Caution in general dictates initial reliance on well-tried remedies. To paraphrase the advice of Polonius to his son Laertes in Shakespeare's *Hamlet*:

Those drugs thou hast, and their adoption tried,
Grapple them to thy soul with hoops of steel;
But do not dull thy palm with entertainment
Of each new-hatch'd, unfledged remedy.

Summary

Stimulant medications provide a rapidly effective treatment of inattentiveness and hyperactivity, the core symptoms of ADHD. Frequent monitoring is required, and for optimal long-term results, medication should be complemented with behavior modification and necessary academic accommodations. Methylphenidate and amphetamine formulations of stimulants are short-acting, intermediate, or extended release. The short-acting preparations have an effect within 15–30 min, a peak effect at 1–2 h, and a duration of action of 3–6 h. Intermediate-acting formulations are released slower, have a peak effect at 4–5 h, and a duration of action of 7–8 h. Extended-release formulations have a biphasic release with peaks at 1–2 and 5–8 h, and duration up to 12 h. A methylphenidate skin patch has a slower onset of action, a plateau release, and duration of 9–10 h, extending for 1–2 h after patch removal.

Each preparation has specific indications and usage, depending on the age of patient, hours of classroom studies, amount of homework, initial or long-term therapy, automobile driving, and physical activities. Failure of one medication requires trial of another, until the optimal therapy with fewest side effects is determined for the individual. The non-stimulant medication, atomoxetine, may be preferred to stimulants in patients with ADHD complicated by tics, seizures, abnormal EEG, or sleep disorders. Antihypertensive medications, clonidine or guanfacine, are preferred in younger children with hyperactive behavior complicated by oppositional behavior, or sleep disorder. Monitoring of cardiac status, weight, and growth is recommended with each of these medications, and cardiac consultation is appropriate in patients with heart murmur and/or family history of acute cardiac failure.

References

Abramowitz AJ, Dulcan MK, et al. ADHD children's responses to stimulant medication and two intensities of a behavioral intervention. *Beha Modif.* 1992;16:193–203.

Ahmann PA, et al. Placebo-controlled evaluation of Ritalin side effects. *Pediatrics.* 1993;91: 1101–1106.

Auci DL, et al. Methylphenidate and the immune system (Letter to the editor). *J Am Acad Child Adolesc Psychiatry.* 1997;36:1015–1016.

Barkley RA, Fischer M, Edelbrock CS, Smallish L. The adolescent outcome of hyperactive children diagnosed by research criteria: I. An 8-year prospective follow-up study. *J Am Acad Child Adolesc Psychiatry.* 1990;29:546–557.

Barkley RA, et al. Attention deficit disorder with and without hyperactivity: Clinical response to three dose levels of methylphenidate. *Pediatrics.* 1991;87:519–531.

Barkley RA, et al. Motor vehicle driving competencies and risks in teens and young adults with attention deficit hyperactivity disorder. *Pediatrics.* 1996;98:1089–1095.

Barrickman LL, et al. Bupropion versus methylphenidate in the treatment of attention-deficit hyperactivity disorder. *J Am Acad Child Adolesc Psychiatry.* 1995;34:649–657.

Biederman J, et al. Diagnostic continuity between child and adolescent ADHD. *J Am Acad Child Adolesc Psychiatry.* 1998;37:305–313.

Biederman J, Swanson JM, Wigal SB, et al. Efficacy and safety of modafinil film-coated tablets in children and adolescents with attention-deficit/hyperactivity disorders: results of a randomized, double-blind, placebo-controlled, flexible-dose study. *Pediatrics.* 2005;116:e777–784.

Biederman J, Krishnan S, Zhang Y, McGough JJ, Findling RL. Efficacy and tolerability of lisdex-amfetamine dimesylate (NRP-104) in children with attention-deficit/hyperactivity disorder: a phase III, multicenter, randomized, double-blind, forced-dose, parallel-group study. *Clin Ther.* 2007;29:450–463.

Bowen J, et al. Stimulant medication and attention-deficit hyperactivity disorder. The child's perspective. *AJDC.* 1991;145:291–295.

Bradley C. The behavior of children receiving Benzedrine. *Am J Psychiatry.* 1937;94:577–585.

Bradley C. Benzedrine and dexedrine in the treatment of children's behavior disorders. *Pediatrics.* 1950;5:24–36.

Brown RT, Amler RW, Freeman WS, et al. Treatment of attention-deficit/hyperactivity disorder: overview of the evidence. *Pediatrics.* 2005;115:e749–757.

Buitelaar JK, Van der Gaag RJ, Swaab-Barneveld H, Kuiper M. Prediction of clinical response to methylphenidate in children with attention-deficit hyperactivity disorder. *J Am Acad Child Adolesc Psychiatry.* 1995;34:1025–1032.

Cantwell DP, Swanson J, Connor DF. Case study: adverse response to clonidine. *J Am Acad Child Adolesc Psychiatry.* 1997;36:539–544.

Casat CD, et al. A double-blind trial of bupropion in children with attention deficit disorder. *Psychopharmacol Bull.* 1987;23:120–122.

Castellanos FX, et al. Controlled stimulant treatment of ADHD and comorbid Tourette's syndrome: effects of stimulant and dose. *J Am Acad Child Adolesc Psychiatry.* 1997;36:58.

Clay TH, et al. Clinical and neuropsychological effects of the novel antidepressant bupropion. *Psychopharmacol Bull.* 1988;24:143–148.

Conners CK, Eisenberg L. The effects of methylphenidate on symptomatology and learning in disturbed children. *Am J Psychiatry.* 1963;120:458–464.

Cox DJ, Merkel RL, Moore M, et al. Relative benefits of stimulant therapy with OROS methylphenidate versus mixed amphetamine salts extended release in improving the driving performance of adolescent drivers with attention-deficit/hyperactivity disorder. *Pediatrics.* 2006;118:e704–e710.

Daviss WB, Patel NC, Robb AS, et al. Clonidine for attention-deficit/hyperactivity disorder: II. ECG changes and adverse events analysis. *J Am Acad Child Adolesc Psychiatry.* 2008;47:189–198.

Denckla MB, Bemporad JR, MacKay MC. Tics following methylphenidate administration. *J Am Med Assoc.* 1976;235:1349–1351.

Douglas VI, et al. Do high doses of stimulants impair flexible thinking in attention-deficit hyperactivity disorder? *J Am Acad Child Adolesc Psychiatry.* 1995;34:877–885.

DuPaul GJ, Rapport MD. Does methylphenidate normalize the classroom performance of children with attention deficit disorder? *J Am Acad Child Adolesc Psychiatry.* 1993;32:190–198.

Dulcan MK. Treatment of children and adolescents. In: RE Hales, SC Yodofsky, JA Talbott (eds). *The American Psychiatric Press Textbook of Psychiatry.* 2nd ed. Washington, DC: American Psychiatric Press; 1994:pp 1209–1250

Dworkin N. Atomoxetine induced electrocardiographic repolarization changes with palpitations in a child. *J Am Acad Child Adolesc Psychiatry.* 2005;44:510.

Feeney DJ, Klykylo WM. Medication-induced seizures (Letter to the editor). *J Am Acad Child Adolesc Psychiatry.* 1997;36:1018–1019.

Feldman H, et al. Methylphenidate in children with seizures and attention-deficit disorder. *AJDC.* 1989;143:1081–1086.

Findling RL, Childress AC, Krishnan S, McGough JJ. Long-term effectiveness and safety of lisdex-amfetamine dimesylate in school-aged children with attention-deficit/hyperactivity disorder. *CNS Spectr*. 2008;13:614–620.

Funk JB, et al. Attention deficit hyperactivity disorder, creativity, and the effects of methylphenidate. *Pediatrics*. 1993;91:816–819.

Gilbert DL, Wang Z, Sallee FR, et al. Dopamine transporter genotype influences the physiological response to medication in ADHD. *Brain*. 2006;129:2038–2046.

Gillberg C, et al. Long-term stimulant treatment of children with attention-deficit hyperactivity disorder symptoms. *Arch Gen Psychiatry*. 1997;54:857–864.

Goldman LS, et al. Diagnosis and treatment of attention-deficit/hyperactivity disorder in children and adolescents. *J Am Med Assoc*. 1998;279:1100–1107.

Greenhill LL, Muniz R, Ball RR, et al. Efficacy and safety of dexmethylphenidate extended-release capsules in children with attention-deficit/hyperactivity disorder. *J Am Acad Child Adolesc Psychiatry*. 2006;45:817–823.

Gross-Tsur V, et al. Epilepsy and attention deficit hyperactivity disorder: Is methylphenidate safe and effective? *J Pediatr*. 1997;130:670–674.

Hammer SA, Pasternak JF, Zecker SG, Trommer BL. Stimulant therapy and seizure risk in children with ADHD. *Pediatr Neurol*. 2001;24:99–102.

Handen BL, et al. Prediction of response to methylphenidate among children with ADHD and mental retardation. *J Am Acad Child Adolesc Psychiatry*. 1994;33:1185–1193.

Hochman JA, et al. Exacerbation of autoimmune hepatitis: another hepatotoxic effect of pemoline therapy. *Pediatrics*. 1998;101:106–108.

Hood J, Baird G, Rankin PM, Isaacs E. Immediate effects of methylphenidate on cognitive attention skills of children with attention-deficit-hyperactivity disorder. *Dev Med Child Neurol*. 2005;47:408–414.

Jensen PS, et al. Collaborative multimodal treatment study of children with ADHD. *Arch Gen Psychiatry*. 1997;54:865–870.

Johnston C, Pelham WE, Hoza J, Sturges J. Psychostimulant rebound in attention deficit disordered boys. *J Am Acad Child Adolesc Psychiatry*. 1988;27:806–810.

Keuthen NJ, et al. Retrospective review of treatment outcome for 63 patients with trichotillomania. *Am J Psychiatry*. 1998;155:560–561.

Kouris S. Methylphenidate-induced obsessive-compulsiveness. *J Am Acad Child Adolesc Psychiatry*. 1998;37:135.

Kratochvil CJ, Wilens TE, Greenhill LL, et al. Effects of long-term atomoxetine treatment for young children with attention-deficit/hyperactivity disorder. *J Am Acad Child Adolesc Psychiatry*. 2006;45:919–927.

Lopez FA, Ginsberg LD, Arnold V. Effect of lisdexamfetmine dimesylate on parent-rated measures in children aged 6 to 12 years with attention-deficit/hyperactivity disorder: a secondary analysis. *Postgrad Med*. 2008;120:89–102.

Malhotra S, Santosh PJ. An open clinical trial of buspirone in children with attention-deficit/hyperactivity disorder. *J Am Acad Child Adolesc Psychiatry*. 1998;37:364–371.

Mannuzza S, et al. Adult psychiatric status of hyperactive boys grown up. *Am J Psychiatry*. 1998;155:493–498.

Marcus SC, Wan GJ, Kemner JE, Olfson M. Continuity of methylphenidate treatment for attention-deficit/hyperactivity disorder. *Arch Pediatr Adolesc Med*. 2005;159:572–578.

Martin A, Scahill L, Vitulano L, King RA. Stimulant use and trichotillomania. *J Am Acad Child Adolesc Psychiatry*. 1998;37:349–350.

McBride MC, et al. Use of Ritalin in the hyperactive patient with seizures controlled by anticonvulsant drugs. *Ann Neurol*. 1986;20:428.

McGough JJ, Biederrman J, Wigal SB, et al. Long-term tolerability and effectiveness of once-daily mixed amphetamine salts (Aderrall XR) in children with ADHD. *J Am Acad Child Adolesc Psychiatry*. 2005;44:530–538.

Millichap JG, et al. Hyperkinetic behavior and learning disorders: III. Battery of neuropsychological tests in controlled trial of methylphenidate. *Am J Dis Child*. 1968;116:235–244.

Millichap JG. Drugs in management of minimal brain dysfunction. *Ann N Y Acad Sci*.
1973;205:321–334.

Millichap JG (Ed). *Learning Disabilities and Related Disorders: Facts and Current Issues*.
Chicago, IL: Year Book Medical Publishers; 1977.

Millichap JG. Usage of CNS stimulants for ADHD by pediatric neurologists. *Ped Neur Briefs*.
1996;10:65.

Millichap JG. *Progress in Pediatric Neurology III*. Chicago, IL: PNB Publishers; 1997a.

Millichap JG. Medication-induced seizures in ADHD. *Ped Neur Briefs*. 1997b;11:63, May.

Millichap MG. Locus of control in children with ADHD. Personal communication. 1998.

Millichap JG, Swisher CN. Ritalin-induced seizures in two children with ADHD. *Ped Neur Briefs*.
1997;11:38, May.

Miyazaki M, Ito H, Saijo T, et al. Favorable response of ADHD with giant SEP to extended-release
valproate. *Brain Dev*. 2006;28:470–472.

Mosholder AD, Gelperin K, Hammad TA, Phelan K, Johann-Liang R. Hallucinations and other
psychotic symptoms associated with the use of attention-deficit/hyperactivity disorder drugs in
children. *Pediatrics*. 2009;123:611–616.

Musten LM, et al. Effects of methylphenidate on preschool children with ADHD: cognitive and
behavioral functions. *J Am Acad Child Adolesc Psychiatry*. 1997;36:1407–1415.

National Institute of Mental Health. Multimodal Treatment Study of ADHD follow-up: 24-
month outcomes of treatment strategies for attention-deficit/hyperactivity disorder. *Pediatrics*.
2004;113:754–761.

Nolan EE, Gadow KD. Children with ADHD and tic disorder and their classmates: behavioral
normalization with methylphenidate. *J Am Acad Child Adolesc Psychiatry*. 1997;36:597–604.

O'Toole K, Abramowitz A, Morris R, Dulcan M. Effects of methylphenidate on attention and
nonverbal learning in children with attention-deficit hyperactivity disorder. *J Am Acad Child
Adolesc Psychiatry*. 1997;36:531–538.

Poulton A. Growth on stimulant medication; clarifying the confusion: a review. *Arch Dis Child*.
2005;90:801–806.

Rajesh AS, Bates G, Wright JGC. Atomoxetine-induced electrocardiogram changes. *Arch Dis
Child*. 2006;91:1023–1024.

Rapport MD, et al. Attention deficit disorder and methylphenidate: Normalization rates, clinical
effectiveness, and response prediction in 76 children. *J Am Acad Child Adolesc Psychiatry*.
1994;33:882–893.

Rapport MD, Denney C. Titrating methylphenidate in children with attention-deficit/hyperactivity
disorder: Is body mass predictive of clinical response? *J Am Acad Child Adolesc Psychiatry*.
1997;36:523–530.

Riggs PD. Approach to treatment of ADHD in adolescents with substance use disorders and
conduct disorder. *J Am Acad Child Adolesc Psychiatry*. 1998;37:331–332.

Rosh JR, et al. Four cases of severe hepatotoxicity associated with pemoline: Possible autoimmune
pathogenesis. *Pediatrics*. 1998;101:921–923.

Safer D, et al. Depression of growth in hyperactive children on stimulant drugs. *N Engl J Med*.
1972;287:217.

Safer DJ, et al. Increased methylphenidate usage for attention deficit disorder in the 1990s.
Pediatrics. 1996;98:1084–1088.

Satterfield JH, Cantwell DP, Schell A, Blaschke T. Growth of hyperactive children treated with
methylphenidate. *Arch Gen Psychiatry*. 1979;36:212–217.

Schachar RJ, et al. Behavioral, situational, and temporal effects of treatment of ADHD with
methylphenidate. *J Am Acad Child Adolesc Psychiatry*. 1997;36:754–763.

Shevell M, Schreiber R. Pemoline-associated hepatic failure: a critical analysis of the literature.
Pediatr Neurol. 1997;16:14–16.

Silva RR, et al. Carbamazepine use in children and adolescents with features of attention-deficit hyperactivity disorder: a meta-analysis. *J Am Acad Child Adolesc Psychiatry*. 1996;35: 352–358.

Silva R, Muniz R, McCague K, Childress A, Brams M, Mao A. Treatment of children with attention-deficit/hyperactivity disorder: Results of a randomized, multicenter, double-blind, crossover study of extended-release D-methylphenidate and D,L-methylphenidate and placebo in a laboratory classroom setting. *Psychopharmacol Bull*. 2008;41:19–33.

Simeon JG, et al. Bupropion effects in attention deficit and conduct disorders. *Can J Psych*. 1986;31:581–585.

Smith BH, et al. Equivalent effects of stimulant treatment for attention-deficit hyperactivity disorder during childhood and adolescence. *J Am Acad Child Adolesc Psychiatry*. 1998;378: 314–321.

Spencer T, et al. Bupropion exacerbates tics in children with attention deficit hyperactivity disorder and Tourette's syndrome. *J Am Acad Child Adolesc Psychiatry*. 1993;32:211–214.

Spencer T, et al. Pharmacotherapy of ADHD reviewed. *J Am Acad Child Adolesc Psychiatry*. 1996;35:409–432.

Spencer TJ, Faraone SV, Biederman J, et al. Does prolonged therapy with long-acting stimulant suppress growth in children with ADHD? *J Am Acad Child Adolesc Psychiatry*. 2006;45: 527–537.

Sprague R, Sleator E. Methylphenidate in hyperkinetic children: Differences in dose effects on learning and social behavior. *Science*. 1977;198:1274–1276.

Stein MA, et al. Methylphenidate dosing: twice daily versus three times daily. *Pediatrics*. 1996;98:748–756.

Swanson JM, et al. Analog classroom assessment of Adderall in children with ADHD. *J Am Acad Child Adolesc Psychiatry*. 1998;37:519–526, May.

Swartwood MO, et al. Methylphenidate effects on EEG, behavior, and performance in boys with ADHD. *Pediatr Neurol*. 1998;18:244–250.

Tannock R, Schachar RJ, Carr RP, Logan GD. Dose response effects of methylphenidate on academic performance and overt behavior in hyperactive children. *Pediatrics*. 1989;84:648–657.

Volkow ND, Fowler JS, Logan J, et al. Effects of modafinil on dopamine and dopamine transporters in the male human brain. *J Am Med Assoc*. 2009;301:1148–1154.

Waring ME, Lapane KL. Overweight in children and adolescents in relation to attention-deficit/hyperactivity disorder: Results from a national sample. *Pediatrics*. 2008;12:e1–e5.

Whalen CK, et al. Does stimulant medication improve the peer status of hyperactive children? *J Consult Clin Psychol*. 1989;57:5435–5449.

Whalen CK, Henker B, et al. Natural social behaviors in hyperactive children: Dose effects of methylphenidate. *J Consult Clin Psychol*. 1987;55:187–193.

Wilens TE, et al. Cardiovascular effects of therapeutic doses of tricyclic antidepressants in children and adolescents. *J Am Acad Child Adolesc Psychiatry*. 1996;35:1491–1501.

Wilens TE, McBurnett K, Bukstein O, et al. Multisite controlled study of OROS methylphenidate in the treatment of adolescents with attention-deficit/hyperactivity disorder. *Arch Pediatr Adolesc Med*. 2006;160:82–90.

Chapter 10
Dietary and Alternative Therapies

Various alternative therapies for ADHD have been offered as substitutes or supplements to medication and behavioral treatments. Some merit a trial in children unresponsive or showing toxic reactions to medications, and others appear to show little advantage except as a placebo. The evaluation of claims for therapies in a disorder such as ADHD, without a single, well-defined cause, is a scientific challenge, requiring controls and appropriate measurement techniques.

Subjective bias or prejudice may be excluded by use of a placebo or control treatment and a double-blind trial. Unfortunately, remedies are often advertised before receiving a rigorous scientific evaluation by recognized experts. Parents, in their efforts to find help, may be confused by enthusiastic claims for novel treatments and may be persuaded to try unproven remedies. Fortunately, most are without physical harm to the child, but many consume time, energy, and finances of the families involved.

Reasons Why Parents May Be Convinced of Benefits from Scientifically Unproven Treatments

Parents are sometimes convinced of the value of a treatment when scientific study has failed to demonstrate effectiveness. The methods of scientific study using groups of children with ADHD may fail to recognize positive effects in individuals. Evaluations by teacher and parent questionnaires may not allow measurement of small responses detected by a mother's intuitive observation. Another reason for a parent's enthusiasm for a certain treatment is the so-called "Hawthorne effect."

In Hawthorne, California, a study of the effect of environmental lighting on workers' performance found that performance improved when the workplace lighting was either brightened or dimmed. Light intensity was not important but the change in environmental lighting had an indirect effect on work habits. Similarly, in a parent's evaluation of new treatments for ADHD, the specific type of therapy may be less important than the attention provided by the treatment.

Examples of the failed scientific study in detection of behavioral changes observed by parents are the response of occasional children to sugar and chocolate

J.G. Millichap, *Attention Deficit Hyperactivity Disorder Handbook*,
DOI 10.1007/978-1-4419-1397-5_10, © Springer Science+Business Media, LLC 2010

deprivation and the omission of dyes in the diet. An example of the Hawthorne effect is the benefit that appears to follow sensory and perceptual motor training programs. Children may improve dramatically after enrollment in these exercises, but their effects on learning and behavior may be indirect (Hynd and Cohen, 1983).

Of all the alternative therapies proposed for the treatment of ADHD, diet and dietary supplements have demanded the most attention and invoked frequent controversy. In the following sections, the claims and facts about diet and behavior will be compared by referral to the current scientific literature and disparate results of controlled investigations.

Diets and Diet Supplements Advocated in the Treatment and Prevention of ADHD and Learning Disorders

A list of the dietary treatments proposed for ADHD and learning disorders includes the following:

- Sugar restricted diet.
- Additive and salicylate-free diet.
- Oligoantigenic diet.
- Ketogenic diet.
- Fatty acid supplements.
- Orthomolecular and megavitamin therapy.

For most of these diets and supplements, both positive and negative results have been reported. It may be concluded that a minority of children is responsive to one or another of the diets, but the demonstration of significant effects in a group of children as a whole may defy the available scientific method.

Evidence for and Against a Sugar-Restricted Diet for ADHD

For. Studies in favor of a sugar-restricted diet include the following:

At Colorado State University, 30 preschool children (20 boys and 10 girls, mean age 5 years 4 months) and 15 elementary school children (6 boys and 9 girls, mean age 7years 2 months) received a breakfast of high sucrose content (50 gm), low sucrose (6 gm), or aspartame (122 mg), randomly selected, 5 days on each, using a double-blind control design. On measures of cognitive function, girls made significantly less errors on a learning task performed 30 min following the low-sugar content breakfast when compared to the high-sugar meal, whereas boys were unaffected. On an Abbreviated Conners Teacher Rating Scale completed before lunch, both boys and girls were more active in behavior after the high sugar meal compared to a low sugar intake. Prior to the study, approximately 50% of the children were considered behaviorally sensitive to sugar, based on parent and teacher questionnaires (Rosen et al., 1988).

At the Children's Hospital, Washington, DC, the adverse effects of sugar in children with ADHD were demonstrated only if the challenge dose of sucrose was taken after a high carbohydrate breakfast. The hyperactive response could be prevented by a high protein breakfast (Conners et al., 1984; Conners, personal communication, 1987).

The beneficial and protective effects of a protein diet are correlated with neuroendocrine changes and blocking of serotonergic effects of sugar on behavior and attention. Diets low in protein and high in carbohydrates cause increased spontaneous activity in animal studies. (Yehuda, 1986, 1987).

At the Schneider Children's Hospital, New York, the effects of sugar in a sample of young hyperactive boys with ADHD were similar to those observed by Conners. Inattention, measured by a continuous performance task, was increased following a sucrose drink given with a breakfast high in carbohydrate, but not after a drink containing aspartame (Wender and Solanto, 1991).

Inattentiveness may be benefited by the restriction of sucrose at the morning meal, by avoidance of a high carbohydrate breakfast, or by providing a protein containing balanced meal.

At Yale University School of Medicine, New Haven, CT, the immediate and delayed (3–5 hours) effects of a glucose load on plasma glucose and epinephrine levels were compared in 25 healthy children and 23 young adults. A late fall in plasma glucose (reactive hypoglycemia) stimulated a rise in epinephrine, twice as high in children compared to adults, and hypoglycemic symptoms (shakiness, sweating, weakness, or rapid pulse) occurred in children but not in adults. A measure of cognitive function by auditory evoked potentials (P300 amplitude) was significantly reduced when glucose levels fell to 75 mg/dl in children but was preserved until the level fell to 54 mg/dl in adults (Jones et al., 1995).

Children are more vulnerable to a glucose load and the effects of hypoglycemia on cognitive function and behavior than are adults. The avoidance of rapidly absorbed glucose or sucrose-containing foods in young children might prevent dict related exacerbations of ADHD. A balanced diet of protein, fat, and complex carbohydrates should limit a sudden fall in glucose levels after a meal, and should avoid symptoms related to the epinephrine hormonal response.

At the University of Pittsburgh School of Medicine, mild hypoglycemia (60 mg/dl) caused a significant decline in performance of a battery of cognitive tests in a study of adolescents with insulin-dependent diabetes mellitus, whereas hyperglycemia had no effect (Gschwend et al., 1995).

This study in diabetics supports the theory that a delayed fall in blood sugar following a high sucrose load can have an adverse effect on learning. A sugar-restricted diet may benefit children with ADHD.

At Otto-von-Guericke University, Magdeburg, Germany, the effects of hypoglycemia on cognition were studied using event-related brain potential (ERP) measures and reaction times. Compared to base-line readings, measures of selective attention, choice of response, and reaction time were delayed during hypoglycemia, and responses were slow to recover after normal blood sugar levels were restored. The frontal cortex, known to be involved in the control of attention, was more highly activated than other brain regions during acute hypoglycemia (Smid et al., 1997).

The electrophysiological approach to the study of effects of sugar levels on learning also demonstrates an adverse effect of hypoglycemia, supporting a possible relation between sugar and symptoms of ADHD.

Against. Studies failing to demonstrate either an adverse effect of sugar or a difference between sugar-containing and sugar-restricted meals were as follows:

At the University of Toronto, Ontario, Canada, the frequency of minor and gross motor behaviors, measured by "actometer" readings and video taped observations, was significantly less in 9–10 year-old normal children after the consumption of a sucrose drink than after a drink containing aspartame. Different responses might occur in ADHD children. Also in this study, measures of associative learning, arithmetic calculation, activity level, social interaction, and mood were unaffected by a drink containing aspartame (Saravis et al., 1990).

At Vanderbilt University, Nashville, TN, 25 normal preschool children (3–5 years of age) and 23 school-age children (6–10 years) described by their parents as sensitive to sugar received a diet high in sucrose or an aspartame substitute for three week periods. Measures of behavior and cognitive performance showed no significant differences between the groups. Neither sucrose nor aspartame caused a worsening of behavior or impairment of learning in normal or alleged sucrose-sensitive children (Wolraich et al., 1994).

It may still be argued that individual children are sensitive to sugar or aspartame but adverse effects are difficult to document by limited trial periods in children selected for specific studies.

Partially for or against response. Some studies provided conflicting results, as follows:

At the National Institute of Mental Health, Bethesda, MD, 18 boys, aged 2–6 years, rated by parents as "sugar responders," and 12 male playmates rated as "nonresponders" received single doses of sucrose, glucose, aspartame, or saccharine in a randomized, double-blind design. Parent and teacher ratings of activity levels and aggression failed to show differences between substances for either the alleged "responders" or "nonresponders." No parent differentiated between sugar and artificial sweetener trials. Whereas acute sugar loading did not increase aggression or activity in preschool children, the daily sucrose intake and total sugar consumption correlated with duration of aggression for the alleged sugar-responsive group (Krnesi et al., 1987).

At the Schneider Children's Hospital, New York, boys with ADHD and oppositional disorder and age-matched control subjects received either sucrose or an aspartame drink with a breakfast high in carbohydrate. Measures of aggressive behavior were unchanged by either sucrose or aspartame, but inattention, measured by a continuous performance task, was exacerbated in the ADHD group following sugar, but not with aspartame (Wender and Solanto, 1991).

It follows that the avoidance of sucrose might benefit inattentiveness in the ADD child.

Effects of Aspartame and Diet Sodas in ADHD Children

The FDA and the manufacturer claim that aspartame (Nutrasweet®) and diet drinks are safe, except for children with phenylketonuria. Despite these claims, consumer groups and some scientists issue warnings of reported side effects and nervous system disorders related to the widespread ingestion of aspartame in dietary beverages and foods.

Researchers at the Departments of Psychiatry and Biostatistics, Washington University Medical School, St Louis, have proposed a link between the increasing rate of brain tumors and the introduction of aspartame in the diet in the 1980s (Olney et al., 1996). A review of earlier studies from equally prestigious universities, and published following peer review in recognized medical journals, has concluded that aspartame can precipitate migraine headaches and exacerbate EEG abnormalities in children with epilepsy (Millichap, 1991, 1994, 1997).

Despite the controversy over the validity of these reports and the lack of hard evidence of adverse effects on learning and behavior, aspartame ingestion in children with ADHD should probably be limited, pending a review of its safety by an unbiased panel of experts. The following are some recent reports of the effects of aspartame in normal and in ADHD children:

Studies failing to support a ban on aspartame in children with ADHD include reports from *Schneider Children's Hospital, New York* (Wender and Solanto, 1991), *Vanderbilt University, Nashville, TN* (Wolraich et al., 1994), and *the University of Toronto, Ontario, Canada* (Saravis et al., 1990).

A study at *Yale University School of Medicine*, showing mixed results in 15 ADD children, found no significant differences between aspartame (single morning doses before school for 2 weeks) and placebo on various measures of cognition, behavior, and monoamine metabolism, but a significant increase in activity level following aspartame based on Teacher Ratings (Shaywitz et al., 1994). Until more evidence is available, specifically in ADHD children, Nutrasweet-containing drinks and foods should probably be restricted in the diets of children with ADHD, epilepsy, or headaches.

Current Medical Opinion of the Additive and Salicylate-Free Diet in ADHD

After sugar, additives and preservatives have attracted the interest of parents of children with ADHD more than most items in the diet. The Feingold additive-free diet was introduced in 1975, with the publication of a book entitled "Why Your Child is Hyperactive." Without documentation by controlled studies, the author claimed success in more than 50% of hyperactive children treated. The enthusiasm generated as a result of premature and widespread publicity stimulated the necessity for Federally organized and supported scientific trials.

Controlled studies in two major universities failed to provide convincing evidence for the effectiveness of the additive-free diet to the extent claimed by

Dr Feingold (Conners et al., 1976; Harley et al., 1978a). Nevertheless, a small sub-set of younger preschool children appeared to respond adversely to additives when presented as a challenge (Harley et al., 1978b). It was concluded that an occasional child might react adversely to dyes and preservatives in the diet and might benefit from their elimination.

The interest in additives in relation to ADHD among parents and neurologists in the United States has waned, but in England, Europe, and Australia, the avoidance of foods containing additives is of widespread concern and their relation to behavior continues to be investigated. In a study of the prevalence of food additive intoler-ance in the UK, 7% of 18,000 respondents to questionnaires reported reactions to additives, and 10% had symptoms related to aspirin. A preponderance of additive-related behavioral and mood reactions occurred in children, boys more than girls (Young et al., 1987).

At the Royal Children's Hospital, Victoria, Australia, of 55 hyperactive chil-dren included in a 6-week open trial of the Feingold diet, 47% showed a placebo response, and 25% were identified as likely reactors to additives (Rowe, 1988). In a larger group of 200 hyperactive children, 150 reported behavioral improvements on a diet free of synthetic colorings. A subsequent double-blind, placebo-controlled, 21 day challenge study of 34 suspected reactors identified 24 with a significant behavioral change that varied in severity with the dose of tartrazine synthetic col-orings. Extreme irritability, restlessness, and sleep disturbance rather than attention deficit were the common behavioral patterns associated with the ingestion of food colorings (Rowe and Rowe, 1994).

The number of reactors to the synthetic dye, tartrazine, identified in this Australian study is significant and contrasts markedly with the isolated cases reported in earlier studies in the United States. Children with ADHD complicated by irritability, restlessness, and sleep disturbance may be benefited by an additive-free diet. The strict DSM criteria for the diagnosis of ADHD and an inappropriate behavioral rating scale, omitting irritability and sleep disturbance, may have failed to identify some reactors to food additives in previous studies of the diet. In Australia and the UK, the Feingold hypothesis is still alive, and in the United States, further interest in the use of the additive free diet may be warranted (Millichap, 1993).

At the University of Southampton, UK, preschool children were subjected to a diet eliminating artificial colorings and benzoate preservatives for one week. In the subsequent 3 weeks they were challenged with artificial coloring and sodium ben-zoate added to the diet or with placebo. Behavior was assessed by a tester and by parents' ratings. Significant reductions in hyperactive behavior were noted during the withdrawal period, and significantly greater increases in hyperactivity occurred during the challenge period, based on parental reports but not by objective testing in the clinic. These effects were not influenced by prior levels of hyperactivity or by atopy (Bateman et al., 2004). Adverse effects of artificial food coloring and ben-zoate preservative on the behavior of 3-year-old children are detectable by parents but not by clinic assessment. This study emphasizes the disparity in parental and scientific evaluation of behavior.

In a further study at *University of Southampton, UK,* involving 3-year-old and 8/9-year-old children, artificial colors or sodium benzoate preservative in the diet resulted in increased hyperactivity (McCann et al., 2007).

Foods Omitted and Foods Permitted in the Feingold, Additive-Free Diet for ADHD

According to the Feingold diet, foods to be avoided included apples, grapes, luncheon meats, sausage, hot dogs, jams, gum, candies, gelatin, cake mixes, oleo-margarine and ice creams, cold drinks and soda pop containing artificial flavors and coloring agents. Medicines containing aspirin were also excluded. Red and orange synthetic dyes were especially suspect, as well as preservatives, BHT and BHA, found in margarine, some breads and cake mixes, and potato chips (Feingold, 1975).

Foods permitted included the following: grapefruit, pears, pineapple, and bananas; beef and lamb; plain bread, selected cereals, milk, eggs, home-made ice cream, and vitamins free of coloring. Labels and packages require checking to avoid offending additives, and a dietician should be consulted to ensure that the caloric content and food items are adequate for growth and metabolism. A parent wishing to follow this diet needs patience, perseverance, and the frequent monitoring by an understanding physician.

Oligoantigenic Diet for ADHD

An oligoantigenic diet is one that eliminates all but a few known sensitizing food antigens or allergens. Foods most commonly found to be allergenic include cow's milk, cheese, wheat cereals, egg, chocolate, nuts, and citrus fruits. Skin tests for allergic reactivity to foods are unreliable, and elimination diets are required to test for specific food intolerances.

Lamb, potato, tapioca, carrots, peas, pears, and sugar are examples of hypoaller-genic foods. After introduction of an oligoantigenic diet, improvements in behavior may be delayed for 10 days to two weeks. Individual foods are then added at weekly intervals and withdrawn if allergic symptoms are reproduced.

A combination of the antigen and additive free (AAF) diet is sometimes advised in suspected additive-reactive and allergy prone children (Millichap, 1986). If improvements in behavior are not evident after three to four weeks, alternative methods of treatment are considered.

At the *Alberta Children's Hospital and Learning Center, Calagary, Canada,* a 4-week trial of an AAF elimination diet in 24 hyperactive preschool boys, aged 3.5–6 years, was associated with significant improvements in behavior in 42% and lesser improvements in 12%, when compared to baseline and placebo-control periods of observation (Kaplan et al., 1989). The diet eliminated artificial colors and flavors, chocolate, monosodium glutamate, preservatives, and caffeine; it was low in sucrose, and dairy-free if an allergy to milk was suspected.

Food Antigen Desensitization

At the Universitatskinderklinik, Munchen, Germany, and the Allergy Unit, London, UK, a controlled trial of intradermal food antigen injections resulted in desensitization and tolerance toward provoking foods in 16 of 20 hyperactive children, compared to 4 of 20 who received placebo injections. After desensitization, children with food-induced ADHD were able to eat the foods previously found to cause reactions, especially chocolate, colorings, cow milk, egg, citrus, wheat, nuts, and cheese (Egger et al., 1992).

    These controlled studies lend support to the theory of food allergies and additives as a potential precipitating cause of ADHD in some patients.

Calming Effect of the Ketogenic Diet in Children with ADHD and Epilepsy

In addition to seizure control, the ketogenic diet has a beneficial effect on hyperactive behavior, attentiveness, and cognitive abilities. Antiepileptic drugs known to impair behavior and learning can often be reduced in dosage. (Millichap, 1994).

Omega-3 Fatty Acids in ADHD and Dyslexia

Studies of fatty acid supplements in the treatment of children and adults with dyslexia and behavior disorders provide interesting but conflicting preliminary results. Low serum levels of docosahexaenoic (DHA) and arachidonic acids are reported in hyperactive children with dyslexia, but treatment with supplements in the form of evening primrose oil had only modest and equivocal effects (Mitchell et al., 1987). In a later study in adults, improvements in dark adaptation and reading ability followed treatment of dyslexics with DHA supplements (Stordy, 1995). The Oxford-Durham study, a randomized, controlled trial of dietary supplementation with omega-3 and omega-6 fatty acids in 117 children with developmental coordination disorder and reading disability, found significant improvements in reading, spelling, and behavior over a 3-month period but no improvement in coordination (Richardson and Montgomery, 2005). A similar study in 75 children and adolescents with ADHD found significant improvements, especially in children with ADD-inattentive subtype, following 6 months treatment with omega-3/6 fatty acids (Johnson et al., 2008).

"Orthomolecular" and Megavitamin Therapy for ADHD and Learning Disorders

The terms orthomolecular psychiatry and megavitamin therapy are now used synonymously to describe a theory and treatment of mental illness. The term orthomolecular, very simply stated, means "right molecule." The concept of orthomolecular therapy was adopted by Nobel Prize winner, Dr Linus Pauling, in 1968. He proposed a treatment of mental disease, principally schizophrenia, using megadoses of niacin (vitamin B3), ascorbic acid (vitamin C), other vitamins, the minerals – zinc and manganese, and cereal-free diets. This combination of nutrients was thought to provide the optimum molecular environment for the mind. The treatment was subsequently advocated for children with hyperactivity, and for mental retardation and Down's syndrome (Cott, 1972). An open trial of Vitamin B complex (Becotin®) in ten children with ADHD failed to demonstrate effects on pre- and post-trial measures of behavior and psychological function. A double-blind controlled study was not considered warranted based on these preliminary results (Millichap, 1986).

Biological subgroups of children with autistic and hyperactive behavior may be amenable to treatment with megavitamins and minerals but the efficacy of orthomolecular therapy has not been confirmed by controlled studies. Furthermore, megadoses of some vitamins are not without danger. For example, pyridoxine (vitamin B6), in doses of 100 mg or above, can cause peripheral neuropathy if continued for prolonged periods (Millichap, 1997).

Mineral and Trace Element Treatment of ADHD

The theory of trace element and mineral deficiency as a cause of ADHD and learning disabilities was proposed on the basis of hair analyses and a report of lower than normal values for several minerals. Caution in the interpretation of hair analyses is important, since environmental and seasonal factors, age, sex, and infection can affect mineral concentrations in hair samples, in addition to dietary factors (Millichap, 1991).

Trace elements such as zinc, copper, manganese, iron, selenium, copper, and fluorine can cause disease either as a result of a deficiency state or when consumption is in excess of normal requirements. Toxicity may result from food additives or adulteration, or from non-prescription medicines. The recognition of symptoms and signs of chronic, low-level trace element exposure is often difficult and the interactions between minerals are poorly understood (Millichap, 1993).

At the Dyslexia Institute, Staines, Middlesex, and the Hornsby Learning Centre, London, UK, an association between dyslexia and low concentrations of zinc in sweat analyses has been demonstrated in a study of 26 children, aged 6–14 years, attending for treatment. Hair analyses showed no differences in zinc concentrations but higher concentrations of copper, lead and cadmium were present, when compared to control normal readers. Measurement of zinc in sweat was a more useful

guide to clinical zinc deficiency than hair or serum analyses. The authors theorize that zinc deficiency in the mother might predispose to developmental dyslexia
(Grant et al., 1988).

Mineral analyses, especially zinc, may be warranted in children with learning
disorders, but the need for adequate controls and appropriate specimen collection
is emphasized. Treatment based on inaccurate measurement techniques may lead to
toxicity.

Zinc Deficiency and ADHD

Researchers at *Technical University, Trabzon, Turkey,* investigated the relationships
between serum free fatty acids (FFA) and zinc in 48 children with ADHD and 45
healthy controls. The mean serum FFA level in the patient group was 0.176 mEq/L
compared to 0.562 mEq/L in controls (P<0.001). The mean serum zinc level in the
patient group was 60.6 mcg/L compared to 105.8 mcg/L in controls (P<0.001). A
statistically significant correlation was found between zinc and FFA levels in the
ADHD group (Bekaroglu et al., 1996). The role of zinc in the etiology of ADHD
warrants further study.

Numerous controlled studies report low zinc levels in serum, red cells, urine,
hair, and nails of children with ADHD compared to normal controls and population norms. Zinc supplementation increased the beneficial effect of methylphenidate
therapy. Positive clinical trials of zinc supplementation in ADHD are from Middle-
East countries (Turkey and Iran), areas with suspected endemic zinc deficiency.
Doses above the recommended upper tolerable limit were used, and a 2 in 3 dropout
rate was reported. The role of zinc in ADHD in US children is unclear, based on
previous studies, and further clinical trials were warranted (Arnold and DiSilvestro,
2005).

Investigators at *Ohio State University, Columbus, OH,* correlated serum zinc levels with ADHD symptom ratings in 48 American children, aged 5–10 years. Median
serum zinc levels at the lowest 30% of the laboratory reference range correlated with
parent-teacher-rated inattention but not with hyperactivity-impulsivity. Zinc levels
are related to inattentive symptoms in children with ADHD, but a causative relationship is unproven, and routine treatment with zinc is not yet warranted (Arnold
et al., 2005).

Iron Deficiency and ADHD

Several studies have shown low serum ferritin and iron storage levels in children
with ADHD, but the role of iron deficiency in the cause of ADHD and benefits of
iron supplementation are unproven. A report of low ferritin levels in children with
cognitive and learning disorders (Halterman et al., 2001) prompted our own investigation of serum ferritin levels in children with ADHD. The mean serum ferritin
level of 39.9 ± 40.6 ng/ml was not different than that of control children without
ADHD, but 18% had levels below 20 ng/mL which was considered abnormal. None
had evidence of iron-deficiency anemia. A comparison of the clinical symptoms

of 12 patients with the lowest serum ferritin levels (<20 ng/mL) and 12 with the highest serum ferritin levels (>60 ng/mL) showed no significant difference in severity or frequency of ADHD and comorbid symptoms or response to medications. In our patient cohort, a causative role for low serum ferritin levels in ADHD is not confirmed (Millichap et al., 2006). Supplemental iron therapy does not provide a substitute for medication in the management of ADHD, but given the positive findings in the following report, additional studies may be indicated to define a possible adjuvant role.

Investigators at *Hopital Robert Debre, Paris*, compared mean serum ferritin levels in 53 children with ADHD, aged 4–14 years, and 27 controls. Mean serum ferritin levels were 23 ng/ml in ADHD children compared to 44 ng/ml in controls ($P<0.001$). Low serum ferritin levels were correlated with more severe general ADHD symptoms measured with Conners' Parent Rating Scale and greater cognitive deficits (Konofal et al., 2004, 2007). Iron supplementation (80 mg/day) was followed after 12 weeks by a significant decrease in symptoms on the Clinical Global Impression-Severity Scale but not when evaluated by the Conners' Parent and Teacher Rating Scales. (Konofal et al., 2008). Further controlled trial may be warranted.

Electroencephalographic Biofeedback (Neurotherapy) in the Treatment of ADHD

Children with hyperactive behavior and attention deficits have a high incidence of abnormal EEGs, and poorly organized alpha-wave activity in the occipital leads is a common finding. Patients can control their alpha-wave activity, and a high production of alpha waves at 8–14 Hz is associated with mental alertness and physical relaxation. This is the basis for alpha-wave conditioning via biofeedback techniques in the treatment of ADHD. The treatment requires subject collaboration and may not be practical as an office therapy for ADHD children.

Investigators at *University of Tubingen, Germany*, studied 23 children with ADHD, aged 8–13 years, who received 30 sessions of self-regulation training of slow cortical potentials. Significant improvement in behavior, attention, and IQ score occurred after training and persisted at 6-month follow-up. Slow cortical potential feedback, if confirmed by controlled studies, may prove a viable treatment option (Strehl et al., 2006).

At the *University of Zurich, Switzerland*, 26 children, mean age 11.1 years, diagnosed with ADHD were assigned to neurofeedback training ($n=14$) or group therapy ($n-12$). Slow cortical potential neurofeedback improved only selected attentional brain functions measured by changes in quantitative EEG at rest. The expected improvement in contingent negative variation mapping was not found (Doehnert et al., 2008).

When guidelines established by the Association for Applied Psychophysiology and Biofeedback are followed, EEG biofeedback is considered to be "probably efficacious" for the treatment of ADHD. Biofeedback is indicated in patients

who are stimulant "nonresponders." Approximately 75% of patients may be benefited, according to published reports, but age is probably a modifying factor
(Monastra, 2005).

Vestibular and Sensory Integrative Therapy for ADHD

Sensory integrative therapy employed by occupational therapists is based on a theory, first proposed by Ayres (1981), and outlined in Lerner (1985), that perception
and learning are dependent on brain stem function and organization and balance of
auditory, visual, and tactile processes. An inadequate sensory integration in the brain
stem is postulated in children with learning disabilities, because of immature postural reactions, poor eye muscle control, and impaired visual orientation and sound
perception. Scientific support for impaired sensory integration and touch perception
in children with ADHD is presented in the following studies:

At the Hebrew University, Jerusalem, Israel, somatosensory evoked potentials
(SEP) and tactile function were tested in 49 ADHD children and 49 controls. ADHD
children performed poorly on tactile perception tests, including finger identification, recognition of numbers traced on the palms, localization of touch stimuli, form
perception, and joint movement. The SEP central components were larger in amplitude in ADHD children compared to controls, supporting the theory of brain cell
hyperactivity in ADHD (Parush et al., 1997).

In models of therapy based on these concepts, vestibular, postural, and tactile
stimulation is thought to improve auditory processing and to benefit auditory language disorders and visual perceptual functioning. The therapy involves swinging,
spinning, and rolling exercises that may stimulate the vestibular system. Posture
and motor development are trained by balance and muscle coordination exercises. The tactile system is stimulated through touching and rubbing skin surfaces.
Occupational therapy involving tactile stimulation may lead to improved sensory
integration and accelerated academic achievement.

Central Auditory Evaluation and Training in ADHD

Central auditory evaluation consists of the standard puretone and speech audiometry
or hearing tests together with special tests. These require the identification of signals
distorted by electronic filtering or presented in competition with speech or noise signals. Information regarding attention, decoding, and planning of auditory processing
is evaluated (Jeanane M Ferre PhD, Oak Park, IL, personal communication).

In children with specific language and learning disabilities, scores on dichotic
listening tasks are impaired, suggesting a lack of ability to integrate auditory and
non-auditory information. Pitch discrimination and auditory pattern recognition
skills may be affected, a function of impaired integration of the two brain hemispheres. Intersensory integration skills measured by competing messages in the

two ears may be impaired in children with auditory-visual integration weakness. Excessive reversals are common with integrative central auditory deficits.

The integration of multiple auditory-language and/or intersensory information is necessary for sight word recognition and spelling. Weakness in these central auditory skills may adversely affect the ability to associate sounds and symbols, a skill needed for reading, spelling, writing, language, and communication.

Methods of remediation of central auditory dysfunction are designed to aid integration and organization of material, using verbal rehearsal and visualization, and word association. Playing a musical instrument has been shown to enhance auditory and visual-spatial integration skills and to improve academic achievement.

Children with ADHD occasionally complain of dizziness or vertigo. A referral to an otolaryngologist or neuro-otologist may uncover a dysfunction of the peripheral and/or central vestibular function. Abnormalities of the electronystagmogram (ENG) and brain stem auditory evoked responses (BAER) are indications for a central auditory evaluation. Treatment for a central auditory dysfunction can benefit learning and language disabilities associated with ADHD.

Scientific Basis for Music in Facilitating Learning and Attention

The perception of music is a complex neurocognitive process involving various neural networks, with some anatomical specificity for the different basic auditory components of music (rhythm, pitch, timbre, and melody). Furthermore, visual cognitive imagery appears to be involved in pitch appreciation. Playing a musical instrument requires the functional integration of both brain hemispheres in addition to finger dexterity and coordination. As my violin teacher, Dr Marvin Ziporyn, correctly commented when I erred on pitch of a chromatic scale, "It's all in the head, not in the fingers!"

At the Wellcome Department of Cognitive Neurology, Institute of Neurology, London, the cerebral functional anatomy of music appreciation was determined in six young, healthy, musically naive, right-handed subjects, using a high resolution PET scanner and oxygen-15 labeled water. Four activation tasks on the same auditory material, consisting of 30 sequences of notes on tapes, were used: (1) identification/familiarity with tunes; (2) attention to pitch task; (3) timbre task; and (4) rhythm task.

Familiarity and recognition of tunes, and the *rhythm* task caused activation mainly in the left hemisphere, whereas the *timbre* task activated the right hemisphere. In contrast to previous studies in brain damaged subjects, *pitch* processing caused activation of the left hemisphere, in proximity to primary visual areas, and reflecting a visual mental imagery (Platel et al., 1997).

At the Department of Physics, University of California, Irvine, the positive effects of music on spatial-temporal reasoning was demonstrated in college students by a special analysis of electroencephalographic recordings. Right frontal and left hemisphere EEG activity was induced by listening to 10 minutes of Mozart (Sonata for

Two Pianos in D Major), and enhancement of spatial-temporal reasoning was carried over in 3 of 7 subjects. Relaxation tapes and minimalist music had no effect (Sarnthein et al., 1998).

In their sophisticated scanning procedure, Platel, Frackowiak and coworkers have demonstrated the functional independence of sub-components of musical expression. The left hemisphere is dominant for rhythm, tune recognition, and pitch perception, while the right hemisphere is involved in timbre or quality of tone perception. The differentiation of pitch requires not only auditory but visual interpretation and mental imagery. Listening to Mozart enhances cortical cerebral activity used in spatial-temporal reasoning.

The positive effects on learning of listening to music and playing an instrument are corroborated by neuroanatomical and electrophysiological studies. Involvement in music can be recommended to children with ADHD and learning disabilities.

Effect of Green Play Settings in Children with ADD

Children with ADD function better after activities in green settings, according to a study at the University of Illinois, Urbana-Champaign (Taylor et al., 2001). Parent ratings of post-activity attention were higher for activities conducted in green outdoor settings than for activities conducted in either built outdoor or indoor settings. The greenness of the play setting was related to symptom severity. ADD symptoms were milder for children with greener play settings. Alternative explanations for these findings were excluded, including contact with nature, social environment, physical activity, types of activity, or timing of medication. The design of the study provided support for a causal interpretation. As proposed in the landscape architecture book, "The School in a Garden" (Millichap and Millichap, 2000), green school yards and classrooms with a view of a natural environment could play an important role in a child's academic progress and emotional well-being.

Summary

Alternative therapies for ADHD are offered as substitutes or supplements to medication and behavioral treatments. Dietary alternatives proposed include sugar restricted, additive and salicylate-free, oligoantigenic, ketogenic, fatty acid supplements, megavitamin and mineral therapies. Evidence is equally divided between studies with probable positive effects and those without or undecided. Electroencephalographic biofeedback, vestibular and sensory integrative therapy, central auditory training, and music are additional forms of therapy sometimes found useful as adjunctive treatment. The benefits of a green environment are also demonstrated in controlled studies. Several alternative therapies are regarded as beneficial by parents of individual children, whereas their effectiveness cannot be demonstrated by placebo-controlled trials in group-studies. In patients who are unresponsive to medication and behavioral therapy, trial of dietary and alternative therapies may be justified in some circumstances.

References

Arnold LE, Bozzolo H, Hollway J, et al. Serum zinc correlates with parent- and teacher-rated inattention in children with attention-deficit/hyperactivity disorder. *J Child Adolesc Psychopharmacol*. 2005;15:628–636.

Arnold LE, DiSilvestro RA. Zinc in attention-deficit/hyperactivity disorder. *J Child Adolesc Psychopharmacol*. 2005;15:619–627.

Ayres A. Sensory Integration and the Child. Los Angeles, CA: Western Psychological Services; 1981.

Bateman B, Warner JO, Hutchinson E, et al. The effects of a double blind, placebo controlled, artificial food colourings and benzoate preservative challenge on hyperactivity in a general popultion sample of preschool children. *Arch Dis Child*. 2004;89:506–511.

Bekaroglu M, Asian Y, Gedik Y, et al. Relationships between serum free fatty acids and zinc, and attention deficit hyperactivity disorder: a research note. *J Child Psychol Psychiatry*. 1996;37:225–227.

Conners CK, et al. Food additives and hyperkinesis. A controlled double-blind experiment. *Pediatrics*. 1976;58:154–166.

Conners CK, et al. The effects of sucrose on children with attention deficit. In: Diet and Behavior. Lubbock, TX: Texas Tech Univ Press; 1984.

Cott A. Megavitamins: the orthomolecular approach to behavioral disorders and learning disabilities. *Acad Ther*. 1972;7:245.

Doehnert M, Brandeis D, Straub M, Steinhausen HC, Drechsler R. Slow cortical potential neurofeedback in attention deficit hyperactivity disorder: is there neurophysiological evidence for specific effects? *J Neural Transm*. 2008;115:1445–1456.

Egger J, et al. Controlled trial of hyposensitization in children with food-induced hyperkinetic syndrome. *Lancet*. 1992;339:1150–1153.

Feingold BF. Why Your Child is Hyperactive. New York: Random House; 1975.

Grant ECG, et al. Zinc deficiency in children with dyslexia: concentrations of zinc and other minerals in sweat and hair. *BMJ*. 1988;296:607–609.

Gschwend S, et al. Effects of acute hyperglycemia on mental efficiency and counterregulatory hormones in adolescents with insulin-dependent diabetes mellitus. *J Pediatr*. 1995;126: 178–184.

Halterman JS, Kaczorowski JM, Aligne CA, Aninger P, Szilagyi PG. Iron deficiency and cognitive achievement among school-aged children and adolescents in the United States. *Pediatrics*. 2001;107:1381–1386.

Harley JP, et al. Hyperkinesis and food additives: testing the Feingold hypothesis. *Pediatrics*. 1978a;61:818–828.

Harley JP, et al. Synthetic food colors and hyperactivity in children. Double-blind challenge experiment. *Pediatrics*. 1978b;62:975–983.

Hynd G, Cohen M. Dyslexia. Neuropsychological Theory, Research, and Clinical Differentiations. New York: Grune and Stratton; 1983.

Johnson M, Ostlund S, Fransson G, Kadesjo B, Gillberg C. Omega-3/omega-6 fatty acids for attention deficit hyperactivity disorder: a randomized placebo – controlled trial in children and adolescents. *J Atten Disord*. 2008; Apr 30 [E-pub ahead of print].

Jones TW, et al. Enhanced adrenomedullary response and increased susceptibility to neuroglycopenia: mechanisms underlying the adverse effects of sugar ingestion in healthy children. *J Pediatr*. 1995;126:171–177.

Kaplan BJ, et al. Dietary replacement in preschool-aged hyperactive boys. *Pediatrics*. 1989; 83:7–17.

Konofal E, Cortese S, Marchand M, Mouren MC, Arnuff J, Lecendreux M. Impact of restless legs syndrome and iron deficiency on attention-deficit/hyperactivity disorder. *Sleep Med.* 2007;8:711–715.

Konofal E, Lecendreux M, Arnulf I, Mouren MC. Iron deficiency in children with attention-deficit/hyperactivity disorder. *Arch Pediatr Adolesc Med.* 2004;158:1113–1115.

Konofal E, Lecendreux M, Deron J, et al. Effects of iron supplementation on attention-deficit/hyperactivity disorder. *Pediatr Neurol.* 2008;38:20–26.

Krnesi MJP, et al. Effects of sugar and aspartame on aggression and activity in children. *Am J Psychiatry.* 1987;144:1487–1490.

Lerner J. Learning Disabilities. Theories, Diagnosis, and Teaching Strategies. 4th ed. Boston, MA: Houghton Mifflin; 1985.

McCann D, Barrett A, Cooper A, et al. Food additives and hyperactive behaviour in 3-year-old and 8/9-year-old children in the community: a randomized, double-blinded, placebo-controlled trial. *Lancet.* 2007;370:1560–1567.

Millichap JG. Nutrition, Diet, and Your Child's Behavior. Springfield, IL: Charles C Thomas; 1986.

Millichap JG. Progress in Pediatric Neurology I, II, & III. Chicago, IL: PNB Publishers; 1991, 1994, & 1997.

Millichap JG. Environmental Poisons in Our Food. Chicago, IL: PNB Publishers; 1993.

Millichap GT, Millichap JG. The School in a Garden. Foundations and Founders of Landscape Architecture. Chicago, IL: PNB Publishers; 2000.

Millichap JG, Yee MM, Davidson SI. Serum ferritin in children with attention-deficit hyperactivity disorder. *Pediatr Neurol.* 2006;34:200–203.

Mitchell EA, et al. Clinical characteristics and serum essential fatty acid levels in hyperactive children. *Clin Pediatr.* 1987;26:406–411.

Monastra VJ. Electroencephalographic biofeedback (neurotherapy) as a treatment for attention deficit hyperactivity disorder: rationale and empirical foundation. *Child Adolesc Psychiatr Clin N Am.* 2005;14:55–82.

Olney JW, et al. Increasing brain tumor rates: is there a link to aspartame? *J Neuropathol Exp Neurol.* 1996;55:1115–1123.

Parush S, et al. Somatosensory functioning in children with attention deficit hyperactivity disorder. *Dev Med Child Neurol.* 1997;39:464–468.

Pauling L. Orthomolecular psychiatry. *Science.* 1968;160:265.

Platel H, et al. The structural components of music perception. A functional anatomical study. *Brain.* 1997;120:229–243.

Richardson AJ, Montgomery P. The Oxford-Durham study: a randomized, controlled trial of dietary supplementation with fatty acids in children with developmental coordination disorder. *Pediatrics.* 2005;115:1360–1366.

Rosen LA, et al. Effects of sugar (sucrose) on children's behavior. *J Consulting Clin Psychol.* 1988;56:583–589.

Rowe KS. Synthetic food colourings and 'hyperactivity': a double-blind crossover study. *Aust Pediatr.* 1988;24:143–147.

Rowe KS, Rowe KJ. Synthetic food coloring and behavior: a doseresponse effect in a double-blind, placebo-controlled, repeated-measures study. *J Pediatr.* 1994;125:691–698.

Saravis S, et al. Aspartame: effects on learning, behavior and mood. *Pediatrics.* 1990;86:75–83.

Sarnthein J, et al. Persistent patterns of brain activity: an EEG coherence study of the positive effect of music on spatial-temporal reasoning. *Neurol Res.* 1998;19:107–116.

Shaywitz BA, et al. Aspartame, behavior, and cognitive function in children with attention deficit disorder. *Pediatrics.* 1994;93:70–75.

Smid HGOM, et al. Differentiation of hypoglycemia induced cognitive impairments. An electrophysiological approach. *Brain.* 1997;120:1041–1056.

Stordy BJ. Benefit of docosahexaenoic acid supplements to dark adaptation in dyslexics. *Lancet.* 1995;346:385.

Strehl U, Leins U, Goth G, Klinger C, Hinterberger T, Birbaumer N. Self-regulation of slow cortical potentials: a new treatment for children with attention-deficit/hyperactivity disorder. *Pediatrics*. 2006;118:e1530–e1540.

Taylor AF, Kuo FE, Sullivan WC. Coping with ADD. The surprising connection to green play settings. *Environ Behav*. 2001;33:54–77.

Wender EH, Solanto MV. Effects of sugar on aggressive and inattentive behavior in children with attention deficit disorder with hyperactivity and normal children. *Pediatrics*. 1991;88:960–966.

Wolraich ML, et al. Behavior and cognitive performance of children unaffected by sucrose or aspartame. *N Engl J Med*. 1994;330:301–307.

Yehuda S. Brain biochemistry and behavior. *Nutr Rev*. 1986;44:1–250, Suppl, May.

Yehuda S. Brain biochemistry and behavior. *Int J Neurosci*. 1987;35:21–36.

Young E, et al. Prevalence of food additive intolerance in the UK. *JRSM*. 1987;21:241–247.

Chapter 11
Prognosis and Prevention

What is the outcome for my child when he or she grows up? is a frequent question asked by parents of ADHD children. "Will he outgrow the ADHD?" "Will he need continued treatment with stimulant medication into adulthood?" "Is there an increased risk of drug abuse in adults with a history of childhood ADHD?" Some of the answers to these questions remain controversial, the outcome being influenced by complicating comorbid disorders and other factors.

Patients referred and treated in a neurology clinic for ADD may have less frequent comorbid disorders and a better outcome than those referred to psychiatry because of prominent symptoms of oppositional and conduct disorders. Many factors, including the cause, severity of symptoms, sex, socio-economic status, intelligence, learning disabilities, quality of education, parental care and emotional climate of the home, as well as medical treatment can influence the outcome. The following answers to questions are derived from group studies, and may not always apply in the prognosis of an individual child.

Do Children Outgrow Symptoms of ADHD?

Medical opinion has changed regarding the outcome of childhood ADHD. Formerly, most pediatricians reassured parents by predicting that hyperactivity would resolve after 12 years of age. Currently, most experts favor a more guarded prognosis, with symptoms persisting to some degree in approximately 50% of ADHD children as they approach adulthood (Barkley, 1990). In some reports, hyperactivity is expected to lessen in adolescence whereas inattentiveness tends to persist. The majority of patients make adjustments for their symptoms, but some experience continuing difficulties requiring treatment, especially those with comorbid psychiatric disorders. Even among psychiatrists, however, opinions vary regarding outcome, a recent study finding that children with uncomplicated ADHD may "outgrow" the disorder.

At the Long Island Jewish Medical Center, New Hyde Park, NY, 85 hyperactive boys with ADHD, referred at an average age of 7 years, were evaluated by psychiatric interview at a mean age of 24 years. ADHD had resolved, only 4% having continuing symptoms. Compared to controls, childhood ADHD subjects were at greater risk of developing antisocial personality disorder and non-alcohol substance abuse (12% versus 3%) as adults. Mood disorders in 4% and anxiety disorders in 2% were not more prevalent than in controls (Mannuzza et al., 1998).

Risk factors for persistence of ADHD into adolescence include the following: (1) a genetic familial history of ADHD; (2) exposure to environmental psychosocial adversity and parent conflict; and (3) comorbidity with conduct, mood and anxiety disorders (Biederman et al., 1996). Risk factors for predicting adult outcome are similar to those for adolescence and also include the following: (1) childhood intelligence estimates; (2) childhood hyperactivity and aggression; (3) child-rearing practices and emotional state of parents; and (4) socio-economic status (Weiss and Hechtman, 1986).

Symptoms Associated with ADHD in Adults

Problems with college education, occupation, or family and social relationships may prompt an adult with ADHD to consult a psychologist or psychiatrist. Common presenting complaints include the following:

- Failure to complete college education because of inability to focus on assignments, impaired concentration, and distractibility;
- Frequent job changes because of poor performance, forgetfulness, and lack of organization;
- Poor social and spousal relationships because of quick temper, impulsiveness, low frustration tolerance, and low self-esteem.

Therapy and counseling can help, but a correct psychiatric diagnosis is essential before specific medication is prescribed. The risk of substance abuse is higher in adults, and bupropion (Wellbutrin) may be a safer choice than amphetamines or methylphenidate.

Samples of hyperactive children followed into adulthood were examined for psychiatric complications, academic achievement, antisocial behavior, problems with employment, and social skills (Weiss and Hechtman, 1986; Barkley, 1990). Compared to controls, children with ADHD are more likely as adults to experience problems in one or all of these areas of functioning. With optimal management, however, the majority of patients make satisfactory adult adjustments and compensations.

The best outcome appears to be associated with milder ADHD symptoms and higher IQ in childhood, together with well-adjusted parents and a stable family environment. The long-term benefits of stimulant medication on outcome are demonstrated in one controlled study (Gillberg et al., 1997), and a collaborative multimodal treatment study (Jensen et al., 1997). Reasons for a decline in treatment of ADHD in adolescence and adulthood are unclear (McCarthy et al., 2009).

Does Stimulant Usage in Childhood Lead to an Increased Risk of Substance or Drug Abuse Among Adolescents and Adults with ADHD?

Children taking methylphenidate or other stimulant medication for ADHD do not appear to abuse stimulants in adolescence or adulthood. In fact, most children will express a desire to discontinue medication as early as possible. Media reports of abuse of stimulants among high school students have involved non-ADHD subjects with potential drug addiction.

Whereas stimulant therapy does not lead to substance use or abuse, the symptoms of ADHD do predispose to increased cigarette smoking and a tendency to alcohol use during adolescence, especially in those with comorbid disorders. Adolescents with ADHD complicated by conduct disorders are two to five times more likely to abuse cigarettes, alcohol, and also marijuana than hyperactive patients without CD or normal adolescents (Gittelman et al., 1985; Barkley, 1990).

Children with ADHD referred to a psychiatric clinic are at increased risk of developing antisocial personality and non-alcoholic substance abuse disorders as grown ups. Substance abuse, mainly marijuana, in adults with a history of ADHD has been reported in 40% of patients with persistent symptoms of ADHD (Biederman et al., 1995), and in 12% of those who have "outgrown" the ADHD by 24 years of age (Mannuzza et al., 1998). Control subjects followed from childhood to 24 years showed a 4% incidence of substance abuse.

Antisocial personality, mood and anxiety disorders increase the risk of substance use and abuse, independent of ADHD. The preferred drugs of abuse are no different among ADHD adults and non-ADHD control subjects, and ADHD patients show no predilection for stimulant abuse. Nonetheless, adult ADHD is often a self-diagnosed condition, and an excuse for job failure, divorce, and spousal abuse. Psychoactive substance use disorder is commonly associated with adult ADHD, and stimulant medication should be used with caution (Shaffer, 1994).

Indications of a Good Prognosis in Childhood ADHD

A favorable outcome, high school graduation, and prospects of a college education might be expected in ADHD children with the following criteria:

- An average or above average IQ;
- Perceptual problems restricted to visual or visuo-motor dysfunctions, and without serious learning disorders;
- Absence of comorbid oppositional and especially, conduct disorders;
- Rapid and sustained response to stimulant medication, alleviating hyperactivity and improving academic achievement and perceptual function;
- Early psychological diagnosis and appropriate remedial education accommodations;

- Well-structured school and supportive home environments that lessen distractibility and improve attention span;
- Understanding parents and teachers who provide successful experiences and encouragement and avoid excessive criticism;
- Environment that bolsters self-confidence and leads to a healthy social and emotional development.

Indications of a Guarded or Poor Prognosis

A favorable outcome is less likely in children with the following complications of ADHD:

- A persistently low average or borderline IQ;
- Global perceptual deficits, auditory and visual;
- Severe dyslexia or other learning disability;
- Poor response or intolerance to stimulant medications;
- Delayed psychological evaluation, and inadequate learning accommodations in school;
- Comorbid oppositional and conduct disorders, impervious to psychotherapeutic intervention.
- Poor structured or emotional home environment.

Reasons Why It Is Difficult to Predict the Outcome of ADHD

ADHD is a heterogeneous syndrome, diverse in etiology and clinical manifestations. Both hereditary and environmental factors are important in the cause and outcome, but generally a specific cause is undetermined or idiopathic. Treatment is symptomatic and multimodal, involving parent, teacher, psychologist, and physician. For the majority, there is no simple or fast cure, and the outcome is determined by a variety of criteria. Studies directed to a more homogeneous cluster of symptoms and signs might lead to closer etiologic diagnoses and more accurate prediction of prognosis.

Preventive Measures Based on Known Potential Causes of ADHD

Several presumptive environmental causes have been linked to ADHD, and the following preventive measures are appropriate:

- Optimal medical attention and nutrition during pregnancy;
- Maternal avoidance of alcohol, nicotine, and drug use, especially cocaine, during pregnancy, birth, and breast feeding;

- Optimal obstetric care and avoidance of brain damage from anoxia and premature birth;
- Prompt pediatric attention to neonatal jaundice, hypoglycemia, febrile illness, convulsions, and thyroid dysfunction;
- Testing and treatment for lead exposure and poisoning in early childhood;
- Educational programs for the prevention of head injuries, accidental drug ingestion, and lead and other poisonings;
- Well-structured and healthy emotional home environment;
- Optimal teacher-pupil ratio in small classrooms that lessens distractibility and facilitates learning.

Summary

Outcome and whether a child will outgrow the symptoms of ADHD are a frequent question of concerned parents. Current medical opinion favors a reduction in degree of hyperactivity in adolescence whereas inattentiveness tends to persist. Risk factors for persistence of ADHD into adolescence include a family history of ADHD, exposure to environmental psychosocial adversity, and comorbidity with conduct, mood and anxiety disorders. Additional factors involved in persistence of ADHD to adulthood are low childhood IQ scores, childhood aggression, emotional instability of parents, and poor socio-economic status.

Symptoms of ADHD predispose to increased cigarette smoking and a tendency to alcohol use in adolescence. Adolescents with ADHD complicated by conduct disorders are more likely to abuse cigarettes, alcohol, and marijuana than do patients without conduct disorder. Stimulant therapy for ADHD in childhood does not predispose to abuse of stimulants or to substance use disorders in adolescence and adulthood. Antisocial personality, mood and anxiety disorders increase the risk of substance use and abuse, independent of ADHD.

Preventive measures to reduce the risk or severity of ADHD in childhood include maternal avoidance of alcohol, nicotine, or drug use during pregnancy and breast feeding; optimal obstetric care to reduce the risk of anoxic brain damage and premature birth; and small classroom environments with academic accommodations that lessen distractibility and facilitate learning.

References

Barkley RA. *Attention-Deficit Hyperactivity Disorder: A Handbook for Diagnosis and Treatment.* New York: Guildford Press; 1990.

Biederman J, et al. Psychoactive substance use disorders in adults with attention deficit hyperactivity disorder (ADHD): effects of ADHD and comorbidity. *Am J Psychiatry.* 1995;152: 1652–1658.

Biederman J, et al. Predictors of persistence and remission of ADHD into adolescence: results from a four-year prospective follow-up study. *J Am Acad Child Adolesc Psychiatry.* 1996;35: 343–351.

Gillberg C, et al. Long-term stimulant treatment of children with attention-deficit hyperactivity disorder symptoms. *Arch Gen Psychiatry*. 1997;54:857–864.

Gittelman R, et al. Hyperactive boys almost grown up. *Arch Gen Psychiatry*. 1985;42:937–947.

Jensen PS, et al. A collaborative multimodal treatment study of children with ADHD. *Arch Gen Psychiatry*. 1997;54:865–870.

Mannuzza S, et al. Adult psychiatric status of hyperactive boys grown up. *Am J Psychiatry*. 1998;155:493–498.

McCarthy S, Asherson P, Coghill D, et al. Attention-deficit hyperactivity disorder: treatment discontinuation in adolescents and young adults. *Brit J Psychiatry*. 2009;194:273–277.

Shaffer D. ADHD in adults. An editorial. *Am J Psychiatry*. 1994;151:633–638.

Weiss G, Hechtman L. *Hyperactive Children Grown Up*. New York: Guildford Press; 1986.

Chapter 12
Management Roles and Research Goals

The child with ADHD benefits from parental care and understanding, a teacher's attention to special educational needs, the psychologist's evaluation and behavior counseling, and a physician's diagnostic skill and medical treatment. Each has an important role in the multimodal management of the problem (MTA, 1999) (see also Chap. 8).

Parent's Role in the Management of the Child with ADHD

The early recognition and optimal management of ADHD may be dependent on the education of the parent in the presenting symptoms and the value of various treatments available for ADHD. The following suggestions are offered regarding a parent's role in the management of ADHD:

- Be alert to the possible development of the syndrome in a young child if a family member has ADHD, the birth is complicated by anoxia or injury, or the early milestones of development are delayed;
- Learn about the early manifestations of ADHD, and consult a physician regarding the necessity for neurological or psychiatric investigations and treatment;
- Obtain a preschool evaluation to determine the correct educational placement and program;
- Consult a psychologist if a learning disability is likely;
- Provide a stable home environment and healthy emotional climate;
- Embrace recommended therapies of proven value used conservatively, and be cautious in acceptance of new and unofficial remedies;
- Join a local parent organization such as CHADD, to keep informed of recent developments and advances in the medical, educational, psychological, and legal fields related to ADHD.

Teacher and Remedial Teacher Roles

- Teachers should be aware of the symptoms and signs of ADHD and alert the parent and physician to the early recognition of the syndrome at preschool or kindergarten levels;

J.G. Millichap, *Attention Deficit Hyperactivity Disorder Handbook*, DOI 10.1007/978-1-4419-1397-5_12, © Springer Science+Business Media, LLC 2010

- Optimum programs of remedial education and academic accommodations should be provided to meet a child's individual needs, and should be based on results of achievement tests and psychological evaluations;
- A teacher's observations and reports regarding a child's response to medications and other therapies are of help to the physician in monitoring progress, and also the recognition of potential side effects of drugs.
- Remedial reading teachers are a necessary adjunct to the teaching staff in providing expert help for dyslexics.

Role of the Psychologist

- The psychologist provides an evaluation of cognitive and behavioral functioning, using quantitative tests of intelligence, reading readiness and ability, arithmetical skills, visual-motor and auditory perception, and ratings of hyperactivity-impulsivity and inattentiveness.
- Comorbid oppositional, conduct, anxiety, and depressive disorders are also noted.
- The psychologist's report is essential to the teacher in determining the correct school placement and remedial program of education, and for the physician's evaluation of the diagnosis and optimal medical treatment.
- A psychologist may be the first to recognize absence seizures in a child who "daydreams" during an examination. By alerting the parent and physician to a potential seizure disorder, an electroencephalogram is expedited and the diagnosis and treatment facilitated. Frequent absence or partial complex seizures may sometimes masquerade as a learning disorder. Tics and obsessive compulsive disorders are often first recognized and reported by the psychologist.
- Family counseling and behavior modification provided by the psychologist are important in the multimodal treatment approach to ADHD.
- Psychologists are not responsible for the prescription of drugs, but their knowledge and expertise in psychopharmacology is valuable to the patient and physician in determining the optimal type and amount of medication required in the individual patient.
- Investigational psychologists have been responsible for much of the behavioral, psychopharmacological, and diet-related research in children with ADHD. Their knowledge of statistical analyses and controlled studies has expanded our scientific understanding and acceptance of treatments and outcome of ADHD. The psychologist's close collaboration with neurologist and psychiatrist is an invaluable asset to the multimodal management team.
- Reports of psychological evaluations intended to aid the overtaxed physician and teacher in the management of the child with ADHD should be concise, emphasizing scores, strengths and weaknesses in comparison with average ability for age. Explanations of the function of tests may be brief while practical academic accommodations are detailed.

Role of Nurse Practitioner and Other Healthcare Providers

The nurse practitioner or physician's assistant may act as physician's associate, collaborating in the evaluation and follow-up treatment of the child with ADHD. A nurse practitioner specializing in pediatric behavioral neurology is an invaluable member of an ADD clinic, coordinating long-term care and prescription refills, and providing advice to parents when requested between scheduled clinic visits. Healthcare providers in some states have authorization to diagnose and treat. The school nurse is a necessary and valuable asset to the treatment of the child with ADHD, supervising the medication administered at lunchtime and reporting side effects.

Occupational, Speech, and Social Worker Services

Occupational therapy is recommended for children with developmental coordination disorder, handwriting problems and sensory integrative disorder. Speech therapy is provided at school and privately for children with receptive and/or expressive dysphasias. School social workers provide counseling for children with oppositional, conduct, and emotional comorbid disorders.

Physician's Role in Research and Improved Management of the Child with ADHD

A number of medical disciplines are involved in the investigation of the causes, diagnostic criteria, and treatment of ADHD:

- Geneticists conduct twin and other studies of hereditary aspects of ADHD, leading to the possible definition of an underlying gene abnormality;
- Pediatric neurologists in collaboration with neuroradiologists are pursuing the MRI volumetric analyses, PET and other brain imaging studies to further define a neuroanatomical basis for ADHD;
- Electrophysiologists are investigating changes in the EEG and evoked potentials during task performance;
- Neurochemists are pursuing the role of neurotransmitters in the cause of ADHD;
- Psychiatrists are periodically changing and refining the symptomatic diagnostic criteria for ADHD and its various subtypes and comorbid disorders;
- Psychopharmacologists are extending trials of methylphenidate and other drugs, observing long-term effects and side effects; The recent introduction of Focalin, a single isomer form of Ritalin, and the novel amphetamines, Adderall® and Vyvanse, are useful additions to medical therapy of ADHD;
- Allergists, mainly in the UK, Europe and Australia, are continuing the investigation of the role of diet and food additives in the cause of ADHD;

- Toxicologists, epidemiologists and neurologists continue research on the effects of lead, iron and zinc on cognition and behavior of children, the frequency of ADHD cases and their distribution;
- Endocrinologists unravel the role of thyroid dysfunction as an infrequent associated factor in ADHD;
- The influence of viral infections during pregnancy and early childhood has received some attention from epidemiologists and pediatric neurologists. Further work on the etiology of ADHD and the development of more specific therapies should be addressed (Millichap, 2008).

Summary

A child with ADHD requires a parent's care, understanding and encouragement; a teacher's attention to special educational needs; the psychologist's evaluation and behavior counseling; a nurse practitioner's medical evaluation and follow-up; and a physician's diagnostic skill and judgment concerning medical treatment. Each has a role in a multimodal method of management, and the cooperation of all parties is essential for the successful monitoring of effective therapies.

References

Millichap JG. Etiological classification of attention-deficit/hyperactivity disorder. *Pediatrics*. 2008;121:e358–e365.
MTA Cooperative Group. Moderators and mediators of treatment response for children with attention-deficit/hyperactivity disorder: the multimodal treatment study of children with ADHD. *Arch Gen Psychiatry*. 1999;56:1088–1096.

Index